M000248201

The Difficult Vaginal Hysterectomy

A Surgical Atlas

Mitchel S. Hoffman
William N. Spellacy

The Difficult Vaginal Hysterectomy

A Surgical Atlas

With 121 Illustrations

Foreword by David H. Nichols

Springer-Verlag
New York Berlin Heidelberg London Paris
Tokyo Hong Kong Barcelona Budapest

Mitchel S. Hoffman
Associate Professor
Department of Obstetrics-Gynecology
University of South Florida
College of Medicine
Suite 529 Harbour Side Medical Tower
Davis Islands
4 Columbia Drive
Tampa, FL 33606
USA

William N. Spellacy
Professor and Chairman
Department of Obstetrics-Gynecology
University of South Florida
College of Medicine
Suite 529 Harbour Side Medical Tower
Davis Islands
4 Columbia Drive
Tampa, FL 33606
USA

Library of Congress Cataloging-in-Publication Data
Hoffman, Mitchel S.
    The difficult vaginal hysterectomy : a surgical atlas / Mitchel S.
Hoffman, William N. Spellacy.
        p.   cm.
    Includes bibliographical references and index.
    ISBN 0-387-94273-4. — ISBN 3-540-94273-4 : DM130.00
    1. Vaginal hysterectomy—Complications—Atlases.   I. Spellacy,
William N., 1934– . II. Title.
    [DNLM: 1. Hysterectomy, Vaginal—atlases. WP 17 H711s 1994]
RG391.H65   1994
618.1'453—dc20
DNLM/DLC
for Library of Congress   94-5703
                                                              CIP

Printed on acid-free paper.

© 1995 by Springer-Verlag New York, Inc.
All rights reserved. This work may not be translated or copied in whole or in part without the written permission of the publisher
(Springer-Verlag New York, Inc., 175 Fifth Avenue, New York, NY 10010, USA), except for brief excerpts in connection with
reviews or scholarly analysis. Use in connection with any form of information storage and retrieval, electronic adaptation, comput-
er software, or by similar or dissimilar methodology now known or hereafter developed is forbidden.
The use of general descriptive names, trade names, trademarks, etc., in this publication, even if the former are not especially identified, is not to be taken as a sign that such names, as understood by the Trade Marks and Merchandise Marks Act, may accordingly
be used freely by anyone.
While the advice and information in this book are believed to be true and accurate at the date of going to press, neither the authors
nor the editors nor the publisher can accept any legal responsibility for any errors or omissions that may be made. The publisher
makes no warranty, express or implied, with respect to the material contained herein.

Production managed by Jim Harbison; manufacturing supervised by Vincent Scelta.
Typeset by Asco Trade Typesetting Ltd., Hong Kong.
Printed and bound by Edwards Brothers, Inc., Ann Arbor, Michigan.
Printed in the United States of America

9 8 7 6 5 4 3 2 1

ISBN 0-387-94273-4 Springer-Verlag New York Berlin Heidelberg
ISBN 3-540-94273-4 Springer-Verlag Berlin Heidelberg New York

This book is dedicated to the memory of Dr. James M. Ingram, our beloved friend, colleague, and extraordinary vaginal surgeon.

Foreword

Knowledge of and experience with the basic technique of vaginal hysterectomy is not universal. Each surgeon must learn to identify and appreciate the dimensions of individual variation in anatomic findings and therefore surgical technical decisions and their execution from one patient to another. Unexpected surgical difficulty can be predicted, but ultimately it is dealt with retrospectively. Skilled practitioners must study the particular patient and her problem comprehensively and allow for such individual variations in findings and technical needs as are necessary to the surgical solution for that patient's problem.

Recognizing these factors, Drs. Hoffman and Spellacy have organized and prepared a comprehensive monograph concerning this very real clinical entity. They have reviewed the experience of contemporary surgeons and blended these recommendations with their own experience in a useful compendium of surgical knowledge about this important subject. Their monograph is recommended not as a replacement for the many other fine surgical texts available to the reader but as a supplement to the surgeon's library. It is for those surgeons who, having mastered the basic techniques, are interested in extending the frontiers of personal knowledge of this provocative subject and safely broadening the indications for effective surgery and reconstruction.

David H. Nichols, M.D., F.A.C.S., F.A.C.O.G.
Harvard University School of Medicine
Massachusetts General Hospital

Acknowledgments

The authors would like to thank Dr. Carol O'Kelly, the artist who did all of the illustrations contained in this book. Her skill, hard work, enthusiasm, and attention to detail are greatly appreciated.

They also wish to thank Lynn Larsen who provided the editorial expertise to make the text finally become readable.

Contents

Foreword   vii
Acknowledgments   ix

1   Vaginal Hysterectomy in Perspective   1
2   Standard Approach   5
3   Management of the Adnexa   23
4   Intraoperative Complications   39
5   Enlarged Uterus   53
6   Lack of Descensus   71
7   Markedly Prolapsed Uterus   81
8   Prior Pelvic Surgery   107
9   Miscellaneous Conditions   117

Index   129

1

Vaginal Hysterectomy in Perspective

The first successful vaginal hysterectomy is reported to have been done by Langenbeck in 1813. During the nineteenth century reports of vaginal hysterectomies accumulated as the techniques became modified and the procedure safer. During the later part of the century a few large series appeared that included enlarged uteri requiring morcellation and patients with significant pelvic inflammatory disease.

At the turn of the century abdominal surgery became safer, and by the early part of the twentieth century abdominal hysterectomy came into widespread use and was championed over vaginal hysterectomy by several leading gynecologic surgeons, including Howard Kelly at Johns Hopkins University. Few additional reports of vaginal hysterectomies appeared until the 1930s, however, when the operation experienced a resurgence. At that time several gynecologic surgeons, including N.S. Heaney, reported their results and pointed to a lower morbidity with the vaginal approach. The operation thus came into widespread use again, with its most common indications being small leiomyomas, abnormal bleeding, and prolapse. The relative advantages and indications for these two approaches became a subject of many papers over the ensuing years, but no large prospective randomized study comparing the two operations has yet been published.

Over time, it was gradually accepted that the gynecologic surgeon should be thoroughly familiar with both abdominal and vaginal approaches to hysterectomy so either could be optimally applied on an individual basis. Since the 1960s about one-third of hysterectomies performed in the United States have been done vaginally.

A review of the recent literature and gynecologic surgery texts suggests that somewhat less emphasis has been placed on the more difficult types of vaginal hysterectomy. It is likely that the excellent results obtained with abdominal hysterectomy have encouraged its use for all but those uteri that could be handled by a straightforward vaginal approach. A few of the recent textbooks have dealt with some of the technically difficult types of vaginal hysterectomy, though not in great detail. A few notable recent studies have shown that complicated vaginal hysterectomies, such as those in patients with previous pelvic surgery or enlarged uteri, are safe and may be advantageous for the patient. In 1986 Kovac reported a series of 902 hysterectomies in which 80% were done vaginally.[1] This remarkable figure was accomplished largely through the skillful transvaginal removal of enlarged uteri. In this study, even the patients who had undergone the complicated transvaginal removal of enlarged uteri experienced less morbidity and a shorter hospital stay than those who had undergone abdominal hysterectomy. The advantages of pursuing a transvaginal approach are even more clear in certain groups of patients, such as those who are obese or otherwise medically compromised, as shown in studies by Pratt[3] and Pitkin.[2] There have even been a few reports of vaginal hysterectomy being done on an outpatient basis in selected patients.

It is clear that vaginal and abdominal hysterectomies are not opposing operations. The approach that best suits the individual patient should be chosen. Abdominal hysterectomy is safe and is clearly the proper approach for dealing with complicated pelvic or intraabdominal pathology. The gynecologic surgeon will, therefore, continue to ask why he or she should struggle to perform a difficult vaginal hysterectomy. From a review of the literature as well as our own experience it is thought that, with all other factors being equal, the vaginal approach clearly results in less morbidity and is associated with a significantly quicker recovery. When the gynecologic surgeon has the appropriate skill, the performance of the technically difficult vaginal hysterectomy is a struggle done at the expense of the uterus and the effort of the surgeon but to the advantage of the patient. The purpose of this book is to serve as a guide to the gynecologic surgeon in the approach to various types of technically difficult vaginal hysterectomies.

References

1. Kovac SR. Intramyometrial coring as an adjunct to vaginal hysterectomy. Obstet Gynecol 67:131–136, 1968

2. Pitkin RM. Vaginal hysterectomy in obese women. Obstet Gynecol 49:567–569, 1977

3. Pratt JH, Daikoku NH. Obesity and vaginal hysterectomy. J Reprod Med 35:945–949, 1990

Suggested Reading

Allen E, Peterson LF. Versatility of vaginal hysterectomy technique. Obstet Gynecol 3:240–247, 1954

Altchek A. Vaginal hysterectomy revisited. Female Patient 16:57–59, 1991

Amirrika H, Evans TN. Ten-year review of hysterectomies: trends, indications, and risks. Am J Obstet Gynecol 134:431–437, 1979

Bolsen B. Study suggests vaginal hysterectomy is safer. JAMA 247:13–19, 1982

Bradford WZ, Bradford WB, Woltz JHE, Brown CW. Experiences with vaginal hysterectomy. Am J Obstet Gynecol 68:540–548, 1954

Browne DS, Frazer MI. Hysterectomy revisited. Aust NZ J Obstet Gynaecol 31:148–152, 1991

Campbell ZB. A report on 2,798 vaginal hysterectomies. Am J Obstet Gynecol 52:598–613, 1946

Carlson KJ, Nichols DH, Schiff I. Indications for hysterectomy. N Engl J Med 328:856–860, 1993

Copenhaver EH. Vaginal hysterectomy: an analysis of indication and complications among 1,000 operations. Am J Obstet Gynecol 84:123–128, 1962

Copenhaver EH. Vaginal hysterectomy past, present and future. Surg Clin North Am 60:437–49, 1980

Coulam CB, Pratt JH. Vaginal hysterectomy: is previous pelvic operation a contraindication? Am J Obstet Gynecol 116:252–260, 1973

Cruikshank SH. Surgical method of identifying the ureters during total vaginal hysterectomy. Obstet Gynecol 67:277–280, 1986

Dicker RC, Greenspan JR, Strauss LT, et al. Complications of abdominal and vaginal hysterectomy among women of reproductive age in the United States: the collaborative review of sterilization. Am J Obstet Gynecol 144:841–848, 1982

Easterday CL, Grimes DA, Riggs JA. Hysterectomy in the United States. Obstet Gynecol 62:203–212, 1983

Falk HC, Bunkin IA. A study of 500 vaginal hysterectomies. Am J Obstet Gynecol 52:623–630, 1946

Gitsch G, Berger E, Tatra G. Trends in thirty years of vaginal hysterectomy. Surg Gynecol Obstet 172:207–210, 1991

Gray LA. Indications, techniques, and complications in vaginal hysterectomy. Obstet Gynecol 28:714–722, 1966

Gray LA. Vaginal Hysterectomy, Charles C Thomas, Springfield, IL, 1955

Harris BA. Vaginal hysterectomy in a community hospital. NY State J Med 76:1304–1307, 1976.

Heaney NS. A report of 565 vaginal hysterectomies performed for benign pelvic disease. Am J Obstet Gynecol 28:751–755, 1934

Ingram JM, Withers RW, Wright HL. The debated indications for vaginal hysterectomy. South Med J 51:869–872, 1958

Ingram JM, Withers RW, Wright HL. Vaginal hysterectomy after previous pelvic surgery. Am J Obstet Gynecol 74:1181–1186, 1957

Isaacs JH. Vaginal hysterectomy. In Sciarra JJ, Droegemueller W (eds). Gynecology and Obstetrics (Vol 1). Lippincott, Philadelphia, 1990, pp 1–10

Isaacs JH. Vaginal surgery today. Female Patient 16:27–31, 1991

Käser O, Iklé FA, Hirsch HA. In Friedman EA (ed). Vaginal hysterectomy and vaginal procedures for descensus. Atlas of Gynecologic Surgery. (2nd ed). Thieme-Stratton, New York, 1985

Kudo R, Yamauchi O, Okazaki T, et al. Vaginal hysterectomy without ligation of the ligaments of the cervix uteri. Surg Gynecol Obstet 170:299–305, 1990

Lash AF. A method for reducing the size of the uterus in vaginal hysterectomy. Am J Obstet Gynecol 42:452–459, 1941

Leventhal ML, Lazarus ML. Total abdominal and vaginal hysterectomy, a comparison. Am J Obstet Gynecol 61:289–299, 1951

Masterson BJ. Manual of Gynecologic Surgery (2nd ed). Springer, New York, 1986, pp 108–121

Mattingly RF, Thompson JD: Telinde's Operative Gynecology (6th ed). Lippincott, Philadelphia, 1985, pp. 548–560

Nichols DH, Randall CL. Vaginal Surgery (3rd ed). Williams & Wilkins, Baltimore, 1989, pp 182–238

Perineau M, Monrozies X, Reme JM. Complications of hysterectomy. Rev Fr Gynecol Obstet 87:120–125, 1992

Pitkin RM. Abdominal hysterectomy in obese women. Obstet Gynecol 142:532–536, 1976

Porges RF. Changing indications for vaginal hysterectomy. Am J Obstet Gynecol 136:153–158, 1980

Porges RF. Vaginal hysterectomy at Bellevue Hospital: an experience in teaching residents, 1963-1967. Obstet Gynecol 35:300–313, 1970

Powers TW, Goodno JA Jr, Harris VD. The outpatient vaginal hysterectomy. Am J Obstet Gynecol 168:1875–1880, 1992

Pratt JH, Gunnlaugsson GH. Vaginal hysterectomy by morcellation. Mayo Clin Proc 45:374–387, 1970

Reiffenstuhl G, Platzer W, Friedman EA (eds). Atlas of Vaginal Surgery: Surgical Anatomy and Technique (Vol 1). Saunders, Philadelphia, 1975, pp 286–329

Reiner IJ. Early discharge after vaginal hysterectomy. Obstet Gynecol 71:416–418, 1988

Sheth S, Malpani A. Vaginal hysterectomy for the management of menstruation in mentally retarded women. Int J Gynaecol Obstet 35:319–321, 1991

Stovall TG, Summitt RL Jr, Bran DF, Ling FW. Outpatient vaginal hysterectomy: a pilot study. Obstet Gynecol 80:145–149, 1992

Wheeless CR Jr. Atlas of Pelvic Surgery (2nd ed). Lea & Febiger, Philadelphia, 1988, pp 241–249

White SC, Watel LJ, Wade ME. Comparison of abdominal and vaginal hysterectomies: a review of 600 operations. Obstet Gynecol 37:530–537, 1971

2

Standard Approach

For some women it is readily apparent that hysterectomy can be accomplished transvaginally. Providing that one adheres to some basic principles, this approach can be used with a variety of techniques. As a prelude to more difficult aspects of vaginal hysterectomy, this chapter describes a general approach to the relatively straightforward case. As is emphasized throughout this text, versatility in techniques rather than a single standard approach is of importance for the vaginal hysterectomy. It provides the surgeon with the adaptability to utilize a surgical approach that is best suited to the individual case. Greater versatility and adaptability of the surgeon are especially important elements in successfully managing the more technically difficult types of vaginal hysterectomy.

Each gynecologic surgeon develops his or her own personal approach to the vaginal hysterectomy. In some situations the gynecologist finds that variations of technique are required to facilitate completion of the hysterectomy. Knowledge of various techniques, along with skill and experience, allows the gynecologic surgeon to complete difficult vaginal hysterectomies. The patient benefits from this experience by a less uncomfortable and more rapid recovery period.

Vaginal hysterectomy is done with the patient in the dorsal lithotomy position. It is the surgeon's responsibility to position the patient carefully to provide optimal exposure for both the surgeon and the assistants and at the same time to avoid nerve injury. Careful examination under anesthesia is the best time to determine if it is reasonable to perform the hysterectomy vaginally. Bony pelvic architecture, uterine size and configuration, and uterine descensus and mobility are the anatomic factors that must be evaluated. The patient's general condition, the indication for the hysterectomy, and other factors also enter into the choice of hysterectomy route. After evaluating these factors, the decision to proceed with a vaginal approach is finally made based on the individual skill and judgment of the gynecologic surgeon.

A hysterectomy begun vaginally occasionally must be completed abdominally. Accordingly, every patient should be informed of this possibility before the start of the procedure so she is not surprised to find an abdominal wound upon awakening. Provided the decision is made in a reasonably timely manner, there are no untoward consequences for the patient. In contrast, the patient probably does not benefit from hours of struggle to remove a uterus vaginally that could have been removed quickly and easily by laparotomy. Abdominal hysterectomy is a safe, well tolerated procedure in most patients. Several disease processes call for an abdominal approach to hysterectomy, and in some patients the surgical anatomy is such that a vaginal hysterectomy would likely result in a prolonged operative struggle with limited exposure, subjecting the patient to an increased risk of hemorrhage, infection, and urinary tract injury. Again, gynecologic surgeons must use their judgment when selecting the best approach for the individual patient.

Before proceeding further, brief mention should be made of the importance of assistance and instruments. Good visualization of the operative field is important for any operation but especially for the difficult vaginal hysterectomy. Ideally, the assistant is a skilled vaginal surgeon as well. Also of significance are the instruments to be used. The pedicle clamps assume the greatest importance when attempting difficult cases. For this purpose the Z-clamp parametrium forceps (Zinnanti Surgical Instruments, Inc., Division of BEI, 21540-B Prairie St., Chatsworth, CA 91311 (800) 223-4740) are useful for two reasons: (1) the pedicles rarely slip from these clamps; and (2) the variation in both angle and length (8.25, 9.5, and 12.0 inches) of these clamps provides great versatility when approaching the various pedicles. Other useful instruments include long, heavy Mayo scissors, Jorghenson scissors, long Allis clamps, a long needle holder, single-tooth tenaculums, a Bovie extender, a weighted speculum with an extra long blade, Heaney right-angle retractors, and a neurosurgery headlight. These instruments are displayed in Figure 2-1.

The examination under anesthesia is an important time to note the presence of genital tract defects or abnormalities. After the pa-

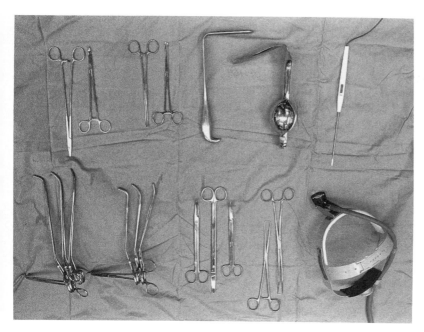

Figure 2-1. Useful instruments that provide versatility for vaginal hysterectomy. *Left to right, top row:* Long and Heaney needle holders, long Allis clamps, Heaney retractor, long-billed weighted speculum, Bovie with extender. *Bottom row:* Long and regular Zeplin pedicle clamps, Jorghenson and long and regular Mayo scissors, single-tooth tenaculums, and neurosurgery headlight.

tient is prepared and draped and the retractors are placed, the cervix is grasped with a tenaculum. Additional important aspects of surgical anatomy are noted at this time. The location of the bladder, posterior cul-de-sac, and rectum, as well as the length, strength, and surgical usability of the uterosacral–cardinal ligament complex are carefully noted. Before proceeding, a Foley catheter is placed in the bladder, the bladder is emptied, and the catheter then clamped. This maneuver allows periodic review of the condition of the urine and bladder drainage.

In the absence of a medical contraindication such as cardiovascular disease, the cervical, paracervical, and submucosal tissues may be infiltrated with a vasospastic solution such as 10 to 20 units of vasopressin in a 50 ml solution or 20 to 30 ml of 1:200,000 epinephrine, which comes as a readily available solution in 0.5% Xylocaine. This step effectively controls "back bleeding" and vaginal mucosal bleeding, and it helps to identify the plane of dissection.

The vaginal hysterectomy then begins with an incision into the cervicovaginal mucosa. The initial incision may be made anterior to, posterior to, or completely circumscribing the cervix. Once started, the correct surgical depth can be readily identified by elevating the mucosa with scissors or a clamp (Fig. 2-2). The full thickness of the mucosal incision may be carried out with scissors, a knife, or cautery. A safe distance from the bladder must be ensured. The posterior mucosa is mobilized until the cul-de-sac peritoneum is identified and entered. The posterior peritoneal incision

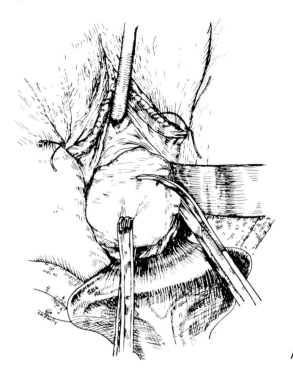

A

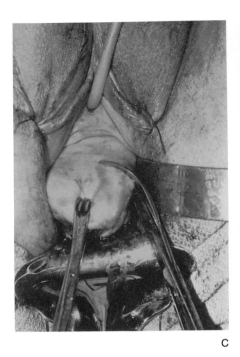

C

Figure 2-2. (A–C) Full-thickness cervicovaginal mucosa being circumscribed with Jorghenson scissors. If a posterior culdotomy has been performed first, the circumcision is completed with the scissors.

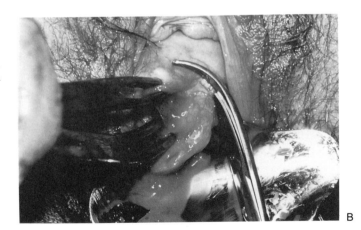

B

is extended to the medial borders of the uterosacral ligaments. Alternatively and more expeditiously, the posterior vaginal fornix may be grasped in the midline at the point of loose reflection, and a direct incision into the peritoneal cavity may be made (Fig. 2-3). If a careful examination under anesthesia has revealed no cul-de-sac abnormalities, this procedure is safe, although there is a small risk of intestinal injury. This method also tends to create a more irregular vaginal cuff.

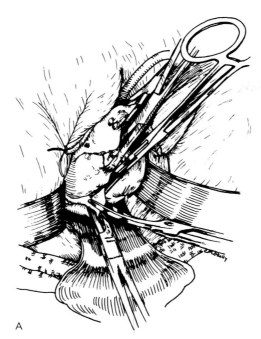

Figure 2-3. (A & B) Posterior vaginal fornix is grasped in midline and a direct incision made into the peritoneal cavity. The fornix is grasped at two sites (one against the back of the cervix) to prevent the peritoneum from folding or slipping away during the incision.

A

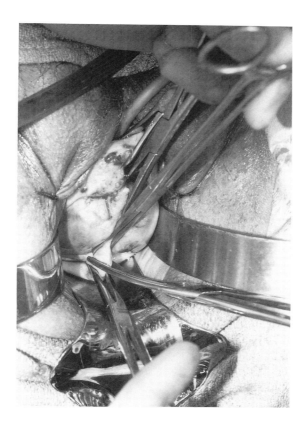

B

Figure 2-4. (A & B)
Supravaginal septum being
breached with long Mayo
scissors.

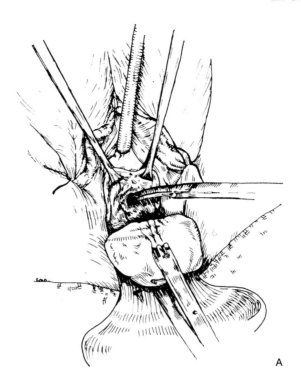

A

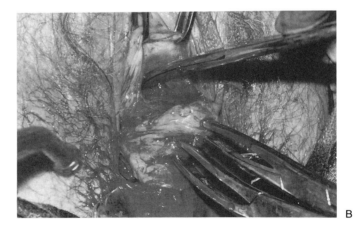

B

Anteriorly, the bladder must be mobilized off the cervix. Some
initial resistance is met for approximately the first 1 to 4 cm (depending on the length of the cervix) by what has been called the
supravaginal septum. This septum is readily breached using a pushing technique with the closed tips of heavy Mayo scissors, with slight
pressure directed against the cervix (Fig. 2-4). Once breached, the
surgeon notes a distinctive sudden loss of resistance. Using the index finger, the space is confirmed and widened. A Heaney retractor

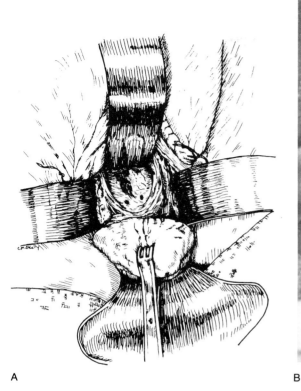

A

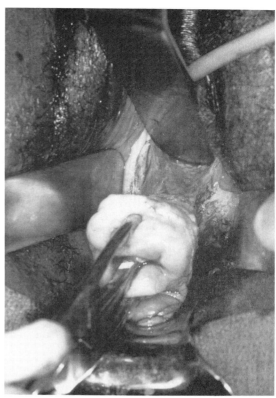

B

Figure 2-5. (A & B) Retractor elevates the bladder, stretching the bladder pillars and exposing the anterior peritoneal fold.

is then placed exposing the anterior peritoneal fold, which causes the bladder pillars to stand out along either side of the retractor (Fig. 2-5). The anterior peritoneal fold usually appears as a clearly demarcated, crescent-shaped line above which is the apparent underside of the peritoneum. The line (actually the point of reflection) is grasped with two long Allis clamps and incised (Fig. 2-6). The peritoneal incision is then extended sharply along the line of reflection, and the Heaney retractor is replaced into the anterior cul-de-sac. Mild traction on this retractor holds the bladder out of the operative field. In addition, the bladder pillars are stretched, further distancing the ureters from the uterus. Sometimes it is necessary to divide several pedicles before accomplishing successful entry into the anterior cul-de-sac.

Figure 2-6. (A–C) Anterior peritoneal fold is grasped with Allis clamps and incised, exposing the anterior cul-de-sac.

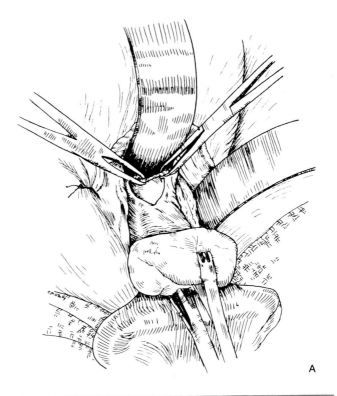

A

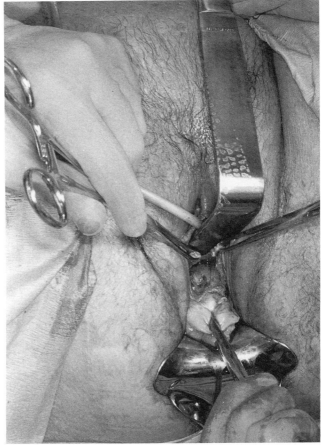

B

Figure 2-6 *Continued*

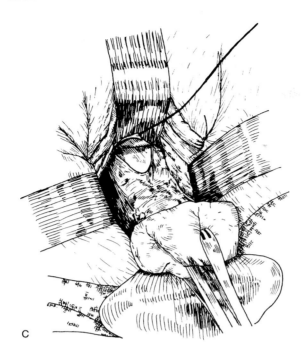

C

Once entry has been gained into the peritoneal cavity above and below the uterus and retractors are placed, the uterosacral–cardinal ligament complex and the bladder pillars stand out well exposed (Fig. 2-5B). With moderate traction on the cervix toward the operator and in the contralateral direction, these ligaments are clamped close to their origin, cut, and ligated (Figs. 2-7, 2-8, 2-9). The first of these pedicles is reattached to the vagina at the time of ligation to support the vaginal vault. The bladder pillars are generally clamped at their base on the cervix with the cardinal ligaments. The ligatures are No. 0 or 1 absorbable suture, and a transfixation type stitch is preferred.

Just above these ligaments at about the level of the uterine isthmus, the uterine arteries are ligated. At this point the anterior and posterior leaves of the broad ligament are brought together in the

Figure 2-7. (A & B) Weighed speculum in the cul-de-sac. Note the uterosacral ligament pedicle with the vaginal mucosa clamped. The tip of the clamp should be close to the most caudal extent of the cardinal ligament. A right-angled clamp (paired with Jorghenson scissors) is excellent for this purpose.

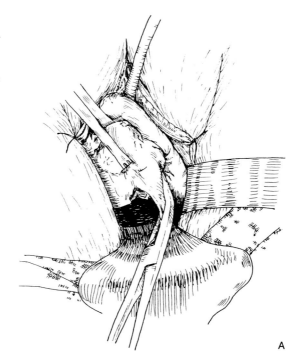

A

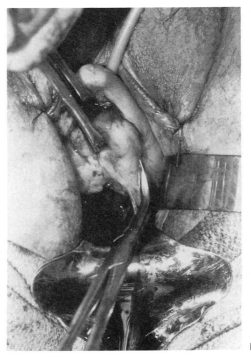

B

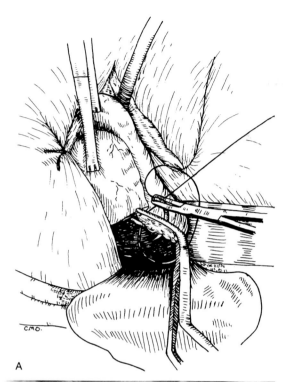

A

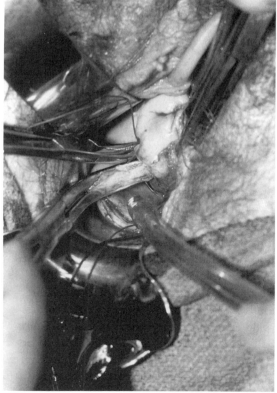

B

Figure 2-8. (A & B) Uterosacral ligament pedicle is cut, and a transfixation suture is being placed.

pedicle (Fig. 2-10). An additional pedicle at the lower portion of the broad ligament may or may not be ligated prior to dealing with the utero-ovarian pedicle.

The utero-ovarian pedicle comprises the utero-ovarian and round ligaments, the fallopian tube, and the utero-ovarian vascular anastomoses. Once this pedicle is divided bilaterally, the uterus is freed for removal. Working cephalad along the lateral aspects of the uterus, the utero-ovarian pedicle is sometimes difficult to access. Exposure to this pedicle is facilitated by applying traction to the anterior or posterior wall of the uterine fundus (Figs. 2-11, 2-12). This maneuver brings the pedicle into and perhaps beyond the vagina, where it can be readily ligated. Care must be exercised when applying uterine traction if only a small amount of tissue remains to support the uterus, as avulsion of these last pedicles is possible. Adnexectomy may be carried out with or as a separate step from hysterectomy. (Management of the adnexae is discussed in Chapter 3.) At this point hemostasis is ensured.

If there appears to be a need for further vaginal vault suspension, a McCall's type culdoplasty stitch is placed with delayed absorbable suture (Fig. 2-13) and held without tying. With the bladder empty, a high purse-string closure of the peritoneal defect is then carried out, further preventing an enterocele (Fig. 2-14), and this stitch is

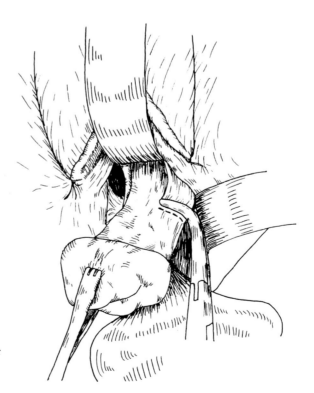

Figure 2-9. Cardinal ligament and base of the bladder pillar are clamped immediately adjacent to the cervix.

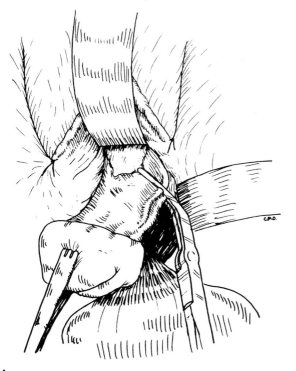

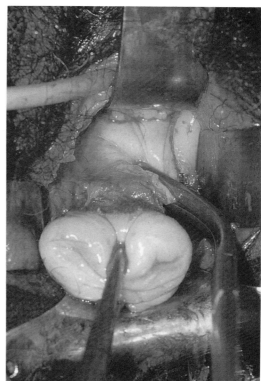

A

B

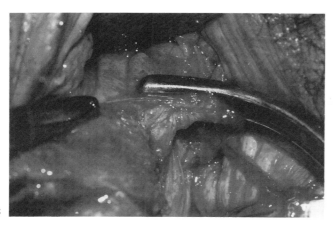

C

Figure 2-10. (A, B) Uterine artery pedicle is clamped, simultaneously connecting the anterior and posterior uterine leaves of the broad ligament. (C) Close-up view.

Figure 2-11. Uterine fundus is "flipped" posteriorly, and the uteroovarian pedicle is clamped.

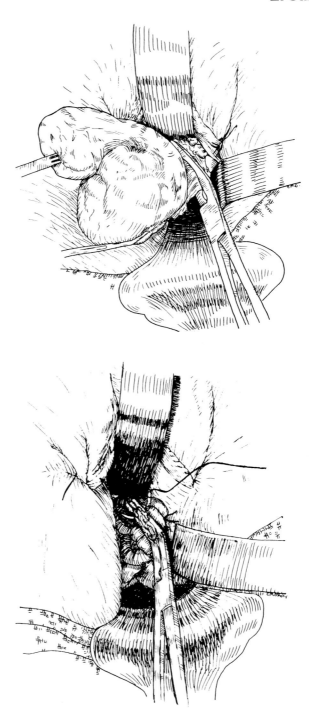

Figure 2-12. Uteroovarian pedicle is cut, freeing the uterus; a free-tie has been placed, a stick-tie is being placed.

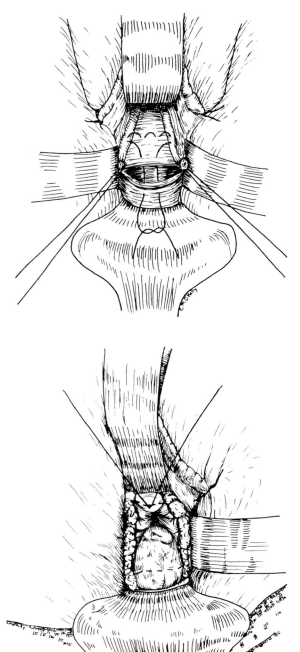

Figure 2-13. Modified McCall's culdoplasty.

Figure 2-14. Purse-string closure of the peritoneal defect.

Figure 2-15. Vaginal mucosal defect is closed vertically.

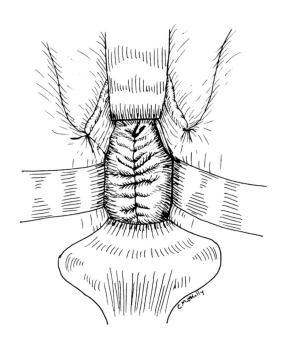

tagged. The vagina is then closed with No. 0 absorbable suture in running interlocking, interrupted, or figure-of-eight stiches, or it is left open with the cut surface edge run with a locking suture technique (Fig. 2-15). Less granulation tissue is induced if polygalactic acid rather than chromic gut suture material is used. A midline vaginal cuff stitch may be tied to the peritoneal closure stitch to close the deadspace. The culdoplasty stitch is then tied. No vaginal packing is placed unless a colporrhaphy is performed. Hemostasis should be sufficient at this point.

Suggested Reading

Campbell ZB. A report on 2,798 vaginal hysterectomies. Am J Obstet Gynecol 52:598–613, 1946

Cruikshank SH, Kovac SR. Anatomic changes of ureter during vaginal hysterectomy. Contemp Obstet Gynecol February:38–53, 1993

Cruikshank SS, Pixley RL. Methods of vaginal cuff closure and preservation of vaginal depth during transvaginal hysterectomy. Obstet Gynecol 70:61–63, 1987

Doderlein A, Kronig S. Die Technik Der Vaginalen Bauchhohlen-Operationen. Leipzig: Verlag Von S Hirzel, 1906

Easterday CL, Grimes DA, Riggs JA. Hysterectomy in the United States. Obstet Gynecol 62:203–212, 1983

Gallup DG, Welham RT. Vaginal hysterectomy by an anterior colpotomy technique. South Med J 69:752–756, 1976

Heaney NS. A report of 565 vaginal hysterectomies performed for benign pelvic disease. Am J Obstet Gynecol 28:751–755, 1934

Julian TM. Vasopressin use during vaginal surgery. Contemp Obstet Gynecol January:82–84, 1993

Kaminski PF, Podezaski ES, Pees RC, et al. The Doderlein vaginal hysterectomy: a useful approach for the neophyte vaginal surgeon. J Gynecol Surg 6:123–128, 1990

Kudo R, Yamauchi O, Okazaki T, et al. Vaginal hysterectomy without ligation of the ligaments of the cervix uteri. Surg Gynecol Obstet 170:299–305, 1990

Leventhal ML, Lazarus ML. Total abdominal and vaginal hysterectomy, a comparison. Am J Obstet Gynecol 61:289–299, 1951

Mattingly RF, Thompson JD. TeLinde's Operative Gynecology (6th ed). Lippincott, Philadelphia, 1985, pp 548–560

Manyonda IT, Welch CR, McWhinney A, Ross LD. The influence of suture material on vaginal vault granulations following abdominal hysterectomy. Br J Obstet Gynecol 97:608–612, 1990

Neuman M, Beller V, Chetrit AB, et al. Prophylactic effect of the open vaginal vault method in reducing febrile morbidity in abdominal hysterectomy. Surg Gynecol Obstet 176:591–593, 1993.

Nichols DH, Randall CL. Vaginal Surgery (34th ed). Williams & Wilkins, Baltimore, 1989, pp 182–238

Pitkin RM. Abdominal hysterectomy in obese women. Obstet Gynecol 142:532–536, 1976

Pitkin RM. Vaginal hysterectomy in obese women. Obstet Gynecol 49:567–569, 1977

Porges RF. Changing indications for vaginal hysterectomy. Am J Obstet Gynecol 136:153–158, 1980

Pratt JH, Daikoku NH. Obesity and vaginal hysterectomy. J Reprod Med 35:945–949, 1990

Sheth SS. Vaginal dimple—A sign of ovarian endometriosis. J Obstet Gynecol 11:292, 1991.

3

Management of the Adnexa

The vaginal approach to hysterectomy is generally confined to patients in whom there is no suspicion of adnexal pathology. Removal of normal or nonadherent ovaries abdominally is straightforward, requiring little additional operative time or blood loss. Transvaginal adnexectomy is often considerably more difficult and not infrequently technically prohibitive. This chapter describes techniques for removal of the adnexa through the vagina. A laparoscopy-assisted technique is described for completeness, and the incidental finding of an ovarian tumor at the time of vaginal hysterectomy is discussed. For the transvaginal approach to adnexectomy, emphasis is placed on good surgical judgment. The surgeon not only should be able to apply a technique of adnexectomy that best suits the individual situation but must also recognize when adnexal removal is likely to be hazardous and best not attempted.

Certain groups of women benefit from prophylactic oophorectomy. One group comprises those over 40 to 45 years of age or who have a strong family history of ovarian cancer. The efficacy of prophylactic oophorectomy for preventing ovarian cancer is a matter of continuing controversy that is beyond the scope of this text. In addition to the possible prevention of cancer, diseases aggravated by ovarian hormones could be averted by oophorectomy at the time of hysterectomy, including endometriosis, breast cancer, polycystic or hyperthecotic ovaries associated with hirsutism, and severe premenstrual syndrome. In addition, the posthysterectomy problems related to ovaries, sometimes termed the retained ovary syndrome, would not occur. The incidence of problems such as cysts related to retained ovaries has been reported to be 2% to 4%. Later removal of ovaries generally requires a laparotomy and is often technically difficult with potentially increased morbidity.

When reasonably normal adnexae are removed during an abdominal hysterectomy, there is little additional effort involved in removing the fallopian tubes along with the ovaries. Transvaginally, however, it is technically more difficult to remove the fallopian tube with the ovary. Excision of the ovary from the mesovarium is more accessible transvaginally than is the fallopian tube and ovary at the level of the infundibulopelvic ligament. The risks of salpingo-oophorectomy are hemorrhage and ureteral injury. There is little danger of injury to the ureter at the level of the mesovarium. Prophylactic salpingectomy has not been emphasized because of the rarity of a primary malignancy developing from this structure. For the surgical management of endometrial carcinoma, complete adnexectomy may be more important. Other conditions, such as old inflammatory complexes, might also call for complete transvaginal adnexectomy (when feasible). The contribution of the fallopian tube to the retained ovary syndrome is uncertain but undoubtedly is a factor. Clearly, individualization of management is warranted based on the surgical anatomy as well as the above factors. For such cases where it is not reasonable to attempt transvaginal removal of the adnexa, attempted removal with such limited exposure risks both hemorrhage and ureteral injury.

Whether to remove the adnexa with or after removal of the uterus is a decision made as the most superior pedicles are approached. The decision is not of great importance except that some time is saved if the adnexa can be readily removed with the uterus. Generally, however, such removal is difficult except in cases of markedly elongated infundibulopelvic ligaments. In most cases it is best to ligate and divide the uterine–adnexal pedicle, remove the uterus, and then attend to the adnexae. Separate ligation and release of the broad and round ligaments from the remainder of the uterine–adnexal pedicle facilitates adnexectomy. One of the ovaries is then grasped with a long Babcock clamp and pulled into the vagina with moderate traction. Oophorectomy or salpingo-oophorectomy is then carried out by one of the following techniques.

Some useful instruments, particularly a long right-angled pedicle clamp, are shown in Figure 3-1. When elongation of the infundibulopelvic ligaments permits, a clamp can be placed above the ovary and fallopian tube (including the round ligament) in a straightforward manner and excision and ligation carried out (Fig. 3-2). This operation is greatly facilitated by separating the round liga-

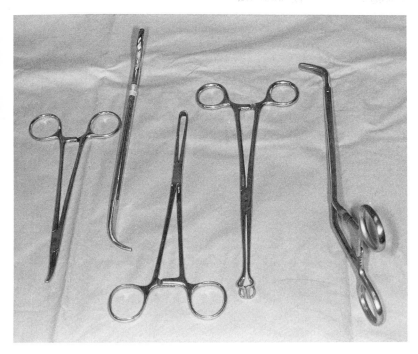

Figure 3-1. Some instruments useful for performing transvaginal adnexectomy. *Left to right:* tonsil, Jorghenson scissors, long Allis clamp, long Babcock clamp, long right-angled Zeplin pedicle clamp.

ment from the remainder of the pedicle (if it was not done during hysterectomy) (Fig. 3-3). Any parauterine broad ligament that was included in the utero-ovarian pedicle may be separated along with the round ligament, or it may be separated by itself. The peritoneum between the round and infundibulopelvic ligaments is then divided, and the retroperitoneal space is developed. After palpating for the ureter, the peritoneum under the infundibulopelvic ligament is then divided. This ligament is now well isolated, allowing both safer and more secure ligation.

Frequently, access to the infundibulopelvic ligaments is inadequate owing to a lack of elongation of these ligaments, as previously discussed. In these cases oophorectomy is often still feasible at the level of the mesovarium. The risk of incomplete removal of the ovary, however, is increased with this procedure. Placing the clamp or free ligature at the base of the mesovarium best enables complete ovarian removal (Fig. 3-4). If the surgical anatomy is such that adnexectomy or oophorectomy cannot be readily accomplished transvaginally, adnexectomy is sometimes accomplished using an endoloop suture (No. 0 plain gut ligature; Ethicon). The endoloop suture is brought around the Babcock clamp and secured either at the origin of the mesovarium or above the adnexa around the infundibulopelvic ligament (Fig. 3-5). Here too it is preferable to separate the round ligament from the remainder of the pedicle before placing the endoloop suture around the infundibulopelvic liga-

Figure 3-2. (A & B) Infundibulopelvic ligament elongated. Adnexectomy is performed in a straight-forward manner by placing a clamp just above the adnexa. Included in the clamp is the round ligament and a portion of the broad ligament.

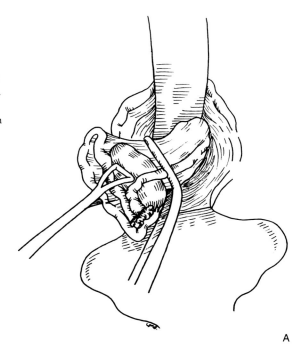

A

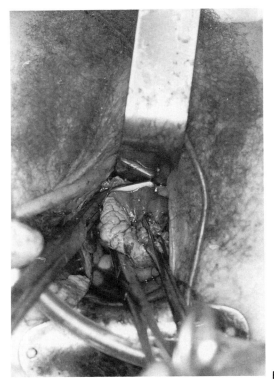

B

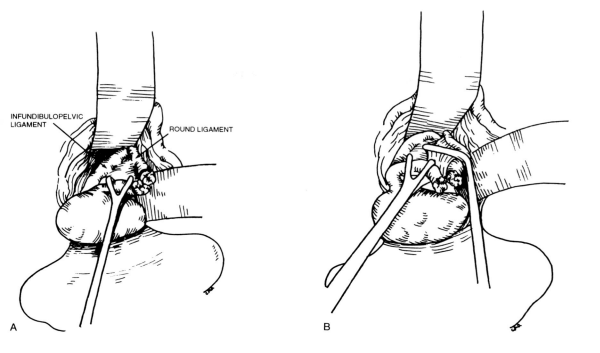

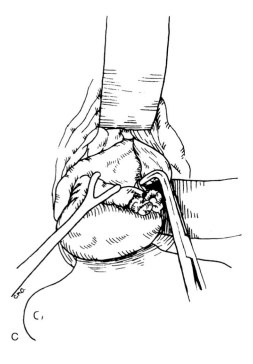

Figure 3-3. Transvaginal adnexectomy is greatly facilitated by separating the round ligament from the remainder of the pedicle. (A) Adnexa is pulled into the vagina with a Babcock clamp. The round ligament extends upward from the pedicle, and the infundibulopelvic ligament extends upward in a medial to lateral direction, with the peritoneum and underlying avascular space between the two. (B) Round ligament and a portion of intervening peritoneum are clamped just above the pedicle. (C & D) Tissue between the clamp and pedicle is cut. (E & F) Intervening peritoneum is undermined and incised. (G & H) Isolated infundibulopelvic ligament is clamped.

Figure 3-3 *Continued*

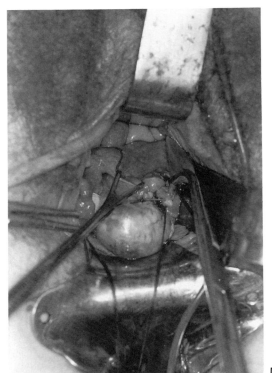

D

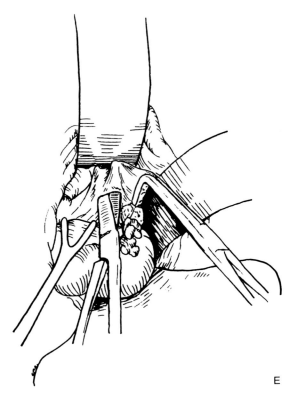

E

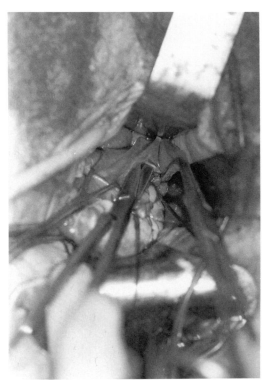

F

Figure 3-3 *Continued*

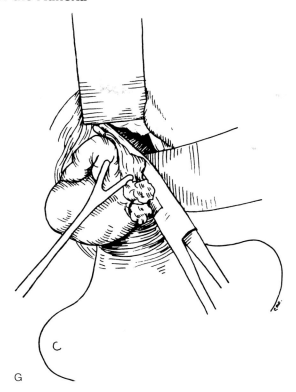

G

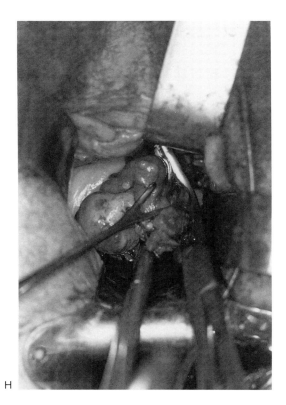

H

Figure 3-4. (A & B) Ovary is pulled into the vagina with a Babcock clamp. A pedicle clamp is placed across the mesovarium.

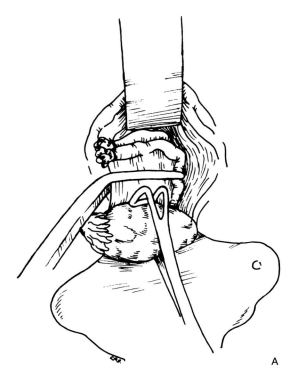

A

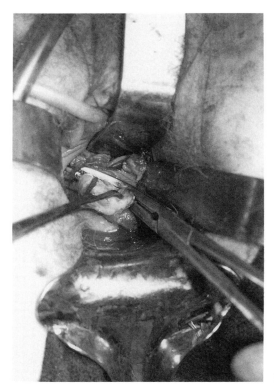

B

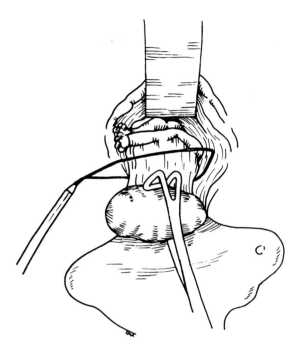

Figure 3-5. Endoloop suture is placed around the mesovarium.

ment. A second endoloop suture can be placed close to the first. The ovary is then excised with right-angle scissors under direct vision while holding the endoloop sutures. A small pedicle of tissue should be left, and great care must be taken during excision not to cut through the endoloop sutures. After excision, traction on these sutures should be avoided.

Laparoscopically Assisted Vaginal Hysterectomy with Bilateral Salpingo-Oophorectomy

Another method that may be used to facilitate removal of the adnexa is a laparoscopically assisted vaginal hysterectomy. With the advent of improved laparoscopic equipment, this method is being described with increasing frequency in the current literature (Table 3-1). A variety of techniques have been described that are not completely covered in this text.

Laparoscopy is performed first, with the patient in low stirrups. Using a multiple-puncture technique, the ovaries may be either completely removed through the laparoscope prior to vaginal hysterectomy or freed up as far as the uterus and removed during vaginal hysterectomy. Our preference has been to free the adnexa as far as its attachments to the uterus and then proceed with vaginal hysterectomy. There is a limited role for this technique: We have used

TABLE 3-1. Laparoscopically assisted vaginal hysterectomy

Reference	No. of pts.	x̄ Operative time (min)	% Laparotomy	% Major complications	x̄ EBL (cc)	x̄ Hospital stay (days)	x̄ Hospital cost (dollars)
1	82	NG	0	0	NG	2.5	12,469
2	68	127	8.8	0	200	3	7,321
4	15	169	0	0	532	3.7	3,926
7	215	114	2	4	86	1.2	NG
8	10	160	0	0	210	2.4	NG
9	75	121	0	0	295	2.4	NG
12	29	120	3.4	10	203	NG	7,905
3[a]	46	191	13	9	210	1.2	NG
6	82	152	2.4	2.4	175	2.6	NG
Total	622	132	3.0	2.7	174	2	9,322

NG = not given; EBL = estimated blood loss.
[a] Stage III and IV endometriosis.

it when there is a strong desire by the patient or a clear indication to remove the ovaries with the uterus and it is anticipated that the anatomic configuration may not readily allow for transvaginal oophorectomy. The performance of a vaginal hysterectomy in patients with a limited degree of descensus may also be facilitated by this technique. Laparoscopy has been reported by Kovac et al. to be useful for determining the best route for hysterectomy in the patient with suspected serious pelvic pathology.[5]

Our technique for laparoscopically assisted vaginal hysterectomy with bilateral salpingo-oophorectomy begins with clear visualization of the infundibulopelvic ligament and the ureter below it. The ureter is visualized through the peritoneum. Lateral to the infundibulopelvic ligament the peritoneum is incised parallel to the ligament for a distance of approximately of 2 to 3 cm, beginning or ending close to the round ligament. The ligament and underlying peritoneum are mobilized medially away from the psoas muscle by blunt dissection of the loose areolar tissue. The peritoneum between the infundibulopelvic ligament and ureter just cephalad to the ovary is then incised for a distance of approximately 2 cm. Klepinger bipolar forceps are used to cauterize the ligament at three separate sites (two proximal and one distal adjacent to the ovary), and the ligament is cut. Alternatively, the Endo GIA (U.S. Surgical Steel) stapling device may be used to staple both sides and divide the ligament simultaneously. After division of the infundibulopelvic ligament, traction is applied to the ovary, and the remaining peritoneum between the ovary and the ureter is incised, thereby freeing the ovary and fallopian tube to the point where they are simply hanging from the attachments to the uterus. The round ligament may then be cauterized and cut and the anterior peritoneal reflection incised. Alternatively, the round ligament may be left intact to "protect" the broad ligament and uterine vessels from avulsion during the vaginal portion of the hysterectomy. The bladder may be mobilized off the cervix using scissors or a "peanut," which is facilitated by fingers or a sponge-stick in the anterior vaginal fornix. An anterior culdotomy may also be performed at this point, but excessive time should not be spent performing additional dissection laparoscopically that can be readily accomplished transvaginally. The identical procedure is performed on the opposite side. At this point the laparoscope may be removed along with the additional puncture instruments with evacuation of the pneumoperitoneum and closure of the small incisions. The patient is placed in sling stirrups, and the operation is completed vaginally. Alternatively, the surgeon may elect to keep the laparoscopic instruments in place in order to irrigate and check for hemostasis immediately after completion of the vaginal procedure.

Unsuspected Ovarian Tumor

Occasionally at surgery the gynecologist discovers an ovarian tumor (Fig. 3-6). When such tumors are large or obviously malignant, a laparotomy is warranted. However, most such tumors are functional cysts less than 6 cm in diameter. One must take great care when handling such ovaries, as bleeding is easily started, potentially forcing surgical intervention. If assessment of the tumor suggests that surgical intervention is warranted and the tumor is accessible, a transvaginal oophorectomy or cystectomy may be performed depending on the individual situation. Although there is a low risk of malignancy, a frozen section should be examined so abdominal exploration can be undertaken at that time if cancer is indeed found.

Preoperative ultrasonography may be helpful in obese women, in

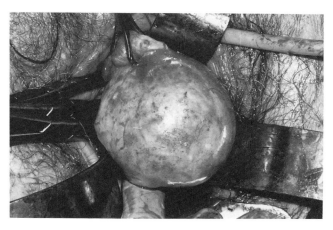

Figure 3-6. Ovarian tumor is encountered immediately after vaginal hysterectomy.

whom pelvic examination is difficult. Ultrasonography should detect ovarian tumors, and the presence of a simple cyst with smooth thin walls almost ensures a benign diagnosis. Other than cystectomy, procedures to facilitate transvaginal removal such as drainage or morcellation are generally not recommended except in highly individualized circumstances. Exceptions may be a medically compromised patient with a large benign-appearing cyst for which drainage, decompression, and removal are easy to complete vaginally. A patient with bilateral ovarian enlargement that is thought to be due to chronic anovulation syndrome might be a candidate for ovarian morcellation to facilitate access to the mesovarium or infundibulo-pelvic ligament.

Whether an individual ovarian tumor can be handled transvaginally depends on several factors, including the size and suspected nature of the tumor, the surgical anatomy of the patient, and the skill of the gynecologist. Careful judgement is the only way to make such a decision.

Summary

Although the adnexae are not easily accessible via the vaginal approach, adnexectomy can frequently be accomplished at the time of vaginal hysterectomy using the described techniques. Reports on transvaginal adnexectomy have established the safety of this procedure. Smale et al. reported 355 cases of vaginal hysterectomy associated with bilateral or unilateral salpingo-oophorectomy.[11] There was one instance of hemorrhage from the ovarian vessels and no recognized ureteral or other serious complications related specifically to removal of the adnexa. In a series of 740 vaginal hysterectomies with attempted oophorectomy, Sheth[10] successfully completed bilateral salpingoophorectomy or oophorectomy transvaginally in 95% of patients. There were no complications directly attributable to the adnexectomies. There are several other reports with similar results. Ideally therefore removal of the adnexa should receive the same consideration regardless of the approach. The gynecologic surgeon's familiarity with the techniques of transvaginal adnexectomy forms the basis for the safe accomplishment of this goal.

References

1. Boike GM, Elfstrand EP, Delpriore G, et al. Laparoscopically assisted hysterectomy in a university hospital: repeat of 82 cases and comparison with abdominal and vaginal hysterectomy. Am J Obstet Gynecol 168:690–701, 1993
2. Daniell JF, Kurtz BR, McTavish G, et al. Laparoscopically assisted

vaginal hysterectomy: the initial Nashville, Tennessee, experience. J Reprod Med 38:537–542, 1993

3. Davis GD, Wolgamott G, Moon J. Laparoscopically assisted vaginal hysterectomy as definitive therapy for stage III and IV endometriosis. J Reprod Med 38:577–586, 1993
4. Howard FM, Sanchez R. A comparison of laparoscopically assisted vaginal hysterectomy and abdominal hysterectomy. J Gynecol Surg 9:83–90, 1993
5. Kovak SR, Cruikshank SH, Raho HF. Laparoscopically-assisted vaginal hysterectomy. J Gynecol Surg 6:185–193, 1990
6. Lee C-L, Soong Y-K. Laparoscopic hysterectomy with the Endo GIA 30 stapler. J Reprod Med 38:582–586, 1993
7. Liu CY. Laparoscopic hysterectomy: report of 215 cases. Gynaecol Endosc 1:73–77, 1992
8. Nezhat F, Nezhat C, Gordon S, Wilkins E. Laparoscopic versus abdominal hysterectomy. J Reprod Med 37:247–250, 1992
9. Padial JG, Sotolongo J, Casey MJ, Johnson C, Osborne NG. Laparoscopy-assisted vaginal hysterectomy: report of seventy-five consecutive cases. J Gynecol Surg 8:81–85, 1992.
10. Sheth SS. The place of oophorectomy at vaginal hysterectomy. Br J Obstet Gynaecol 98:662–666, 1991
11. Smale LE, Smale ML, Wilkening RL, Mundy CF, Ewing TL. Salpingo-oophorectomy at the time of vaginal hysterectomy. Am J Obstet Gynecol 131:122–128, 1978
12. Summitt RL Jr, Stovall TG, Lipscomb GH, Ling FW. Randomized comparison of laparoscopic-assisted vaginal hysterectomy versus standard vaginal hysterectomy in an outpatient setting. In Abstracts of the 40th Annual Meeting of ACOG, 1992

Suggested Reading

Baggish MS. The most expensive hysterectomy [editorial]. J Gynecol Surg 8:57–58, 1992

Campbell ZB. A report on 2,798 vaginal hysterectomies. Am J Obstet Gynecol 52:598–613, 1946

Capen CV, Irwin H, Magrina J, Masterson BJ. Vaginal removal of the ovaries in association with vaginal hysterectomy. J Reprod Med 28:591, 1983

Christ JE, Lotze EE. The residual ovary syndrome. Obstet Gynecol 46: 551–556, 1975

Cruikshank SH. Surgical method of identifying the ureters during total vaginal hysterectomy. Obstet Gynecol 67:277–280, 1986

Daniell JF, Kurtz BR, Lee J-Y. Laparoscopic oophorectomy: comparative study of ligatures, bipolar coagulation, and automatic stapling devices. Obstet Gynecol 80:325–328, 1992

DeNeff JL, Hollenbeck ZJR. The fate of ovaries preserved at the time of hysterectomy. Am J Obstet Gynecol 96:1088–1097, 1967

Donnez JS, Nisolle M. Laparoscopic supracervical (subtotal) hysterectomy (LASH). J Gynecol Surg 9:91–94, 1993

Finazzo MS, Hoffman MS, Roberts WS, Cavanagh DM. Previous pelvic surgery in patients with ovarian cancer. South Med J 81:1518–1520, 1988

Funt MI, Benigno BB, Thompson JD. The residual adnexa: asset or liability? Am J Obstet Gynecol 129:251–254, 1977

Heaney NS. A report of 565 vaginal hysterectomies performed for benign pelvic disease. Am J Obstet Gynecol 28:751–755, 1934

Hoffman MS. Transvaginal removal of ovaries at the time of transvaginal hysterectomy utilizing the endoloop suture. Am J Obstet Gynecol 165:407–408, 1991

Hughes CL Jr, Wall LL, Creasman WT. Reproductive hormone levels in gynecologic oncology patients undergoing surgical castration after spontaneous menopause. Gynecol Oncol 40:42–45, 1991

Kudo R, Yamauchi O, Okazaki T, et al. Vaginal hysterectomy without ligation of the ligaments of the cervix uteri. Surg Gynecol Obstet 170:299–305, 1990

Liu CY. Laparoscopic hysterectomy: a review of 72 cases. J Reprod Med 37:351–354, 1992

Mattingly RF, Thompson JD. TeLinde's Operative Gynecology (6th ed). Lippincott, Philadelphia, 1985, pp 548–560

McCarus SD. Laparoscopically-assisted vaginal hysterectomy. Female Patient. 17:98–102, 1992

McKenzie LL. On discussion of the frequency of oophorectomy at the time of hysterectomy. Am J Obstet Gynecol 100:724–726, 1968

Mikuta JM. Unexpected ovarian tumor discovered at vaginal hysterectomy. In Nichols DH, ed. Clinical Problems, Injuries, and Complications of Gynecologic Surgery (2nd ed). Williams & Wilkins, Baltimore, 1988, pp 41–42

Minelli L, Angiolillo M, Caione C. Laparoscopically assisted vaginal hysterectomy. Endoscopy 23:64–66, 1991

Nezhat C, Nezhat F, Silfen SL. Laparoscopic hysterectomy and bilateral salpingo-oophorectomy using multifire GIA surgical stapler. J Gynecol Surg 6:287–288, 1990.

Nezhat F, Nezhat C, Silfen SL. Videolaseroscopy for oophorectomy. Am J Obstet Gynecol 165:1323–1330, 1991

Nichols DH, Randall CL. Vaginal Surgery (3rd ed). Williams & Wilkins, Baltimore, 1989, pp 182–238

Pitkin RM. Operative laparoscopy: surgical advance or technical gimmick? Obstet Gynecol 79:441–442, 1992

Porges RF. Vaginal hysterectomy at Bellevue Hospital: an experience in teaching residents, 1963–1967. Obstet Gynecol 35:300–313, 1970

Pratt JH, Daikoku NH. Obesity and vaginal hysterectomy. J Reprod Med 35:945–949, 1990

Reich H, DeCapria J, McGlynn F. Laparoscopic hysterectomy. J Gynecol Surg 5:213–215, 1989

Schwartz RO. Complications of laparoscopic hysterectomy. Obstet Gynecol 81:1022–1024, 1993

Sightler SE, Boike GM, Estape RE, Averette HE. Ovarian cancer in women with prior hysterectomy: 14 year experience at the University of Miami. Obstet Gynecol 78:681–684, 1991

Speroff T, Dawson NV, Speroff L, Haber RJ. A risk-benefit analysis of elective bilateral oophorectomy: effect of changes in compliance with estrogen therapy on outcome. Am J Obstet Gynecol 164:165–174, 1991

Tadir Y. Laparoscopic hysterectomy: reinventing the wheel? Am J Obstet Gynecol 167:296–297, 1992

Tadir Y, Fisch B. Operative laparoscopy: a challenge for general gynecology? Am J Obstet Gynecol 169:7–12, 1993

Tasche LW. 1700 vaginal hysterectomies in a general surgical practice. Minn Med 51:1705–1711, 1968

4

Intraoperative Complications

Significant intraoperative complications are an infrequent occurrence during vaginal hysterectomy. It is that very infrequency that catches the surgeon off guard and creates an uncertainty about how to proceed. The relatively limited exposure afforded during vaginal surgery compounds the uncertainty of the surgeon and increases the difficulty of managing certain complications. This chapter discusses the prevention, recognition, and management of the more common intraoperative complications that occur during vaginal hysterectomy. With proper attention to detail, most complications can be recognized and effectively managed transvaginally. Cystoscopy is a useful adjuvant in the armamentarium of the gynecologic surgeon, and familiarity with and liberal use of this procedure are encouraged. For complicated urologic injuries (ureteral, bladder base), one should not hesitate to obtain help from a urologist.

Significant intraoperative complications are uncommon during vaginal hysterectomy. Table 4-1 lists the incidence of intraoperative complications generally reported to occur during vaginal hysterectomy; the data were generated from 15 combined series totaling 24,921 patients.

TABLE 4-1. Summary of intraoperative complications in the literature

Complication	Occurrence[a] (%)
Bladder laceration	0.35
Rectal laceration	0.07
Bleeding requiring laparotomy	0.05
Ureteral injury	0.005
Other intestinal injury	0.005

[a] Based on 15 combined series totaling 24,921 patients (references 1–15).

Bladder Laceration

Laceration of the bladder is the most common complication with a reported incidence ranging from 0% to 0.5%. This injury generally occurs as the surgeon attempts to gain entry into the anterior cul-de-sac (Fig. 4-1). The laceration is usually small, midline, and in the posterior fundus of the bladder above the interureteric ridge. The ureteral orifices are usually a reasonably safe distance from and distal to the entry.

Certain conditions predispose to this injury, including endometriosis, prior cesarean section, and prior pelvic inflammatory disease. The most important aspect of managing this injury is prompt recognition. When the laceration is recognized intraoperatively, it can be repaired with minimal subsequent morbidity and a high rate of success. Prevention of this injury is based primarily on proper surgical technique and is discussed further in Chapter 8.

Several methods have been recommended to help enable the surgeon to recognize a bladder injury intraoperatively. If dissection toward the anterior cul-de-sac has been apparently misdirected or is unusually difficult, the surgeon may have a high index of suspicion that a bladder injury has occurred. In such circumstances it is a simple matter to test the integrity of the bladder with a dilute methylene blue solution. With this approach, however, an unsuspected occult injury would go undetected initially. Occasionally a bladder injury is detected when the surgeon notes urine in the operative field. After emptying the bladder at the start of the procedure, the Foley catheter can be clamped, allowing accumulation of a small amount of urine in the bladder. An incidental entry into the bladder would then be noted by the immediate escape of urine into the operative field. It may be made even more obvious by placing a small amount of sterile milk or dilute methylene blue solution into the bladder at the start of the vaginal hysterectomy. If the urine becomes grossly bloody, a laceration should be sought.

Once recognized, repair of the injury is generally relatively simple and straightforward, and the repair may be carried out as soon as

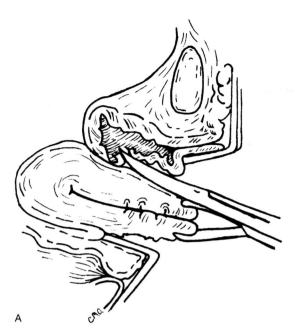

A

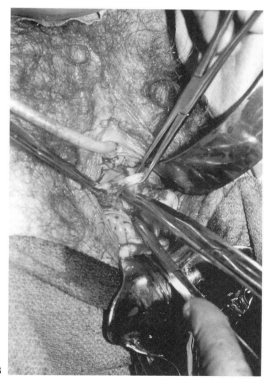

B

Figure 4-1. (A & B) Dissection of the supravaginal septum misdirected into the bladder.

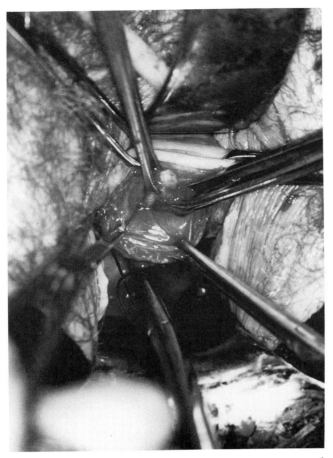

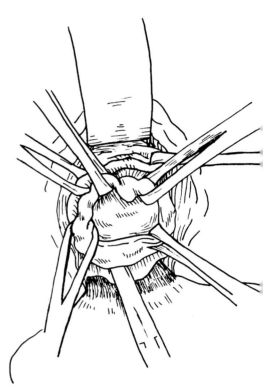

A

Figure 4-2. (A & B) Edges
of bladder laceration have
been completely exposed and
are held with Allis clamps.

the injury is identified. However, entry should at least be gained
into the anterior cul-de-sac before the repair, as cystotomy may facilitate it. It is often easier to complete the vaginal hysterectomy, ensure hemostasis, and then return to the repair. The first and most
important step in the repair is adequate and complete exposure of
the laceration (Fig. 4-2), which is accomplished by gently grasping
what are considered to be the two corners of the laceration with
long Allis clamps. The bladder mucosa should be visualized around
the entire hole. It is sometimes necessary to further mobilize the
injured portion of the bladder from the surrounding soft tissues to
ensure proper exposure and good closure. Starting and ending beyond the corners, the full thickness of the laceration is closed with
a running stitch of 3-0 chromic suture (Fig. 4-3A). There should be

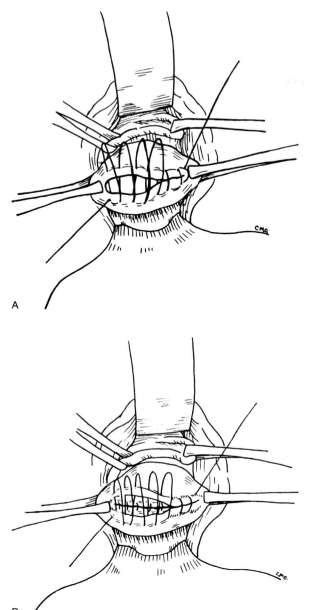

Figure 4-3. (A) First layer of closure of the bladder laceration has been completed. (B) Suture line of the first layer of closure is being imbricated with a second layer of suture placed in the bladder muscularis.

A

B

only enough tension on the suture to approximate the edges. A second layer of 3-0 chromic or delayed absorbable interrupted or running suture is placed in the muscularis so as to imbricate the first layer (Fig. 4-3B). Again these sutures should approximate only. The closure may be tested for water tightness at this point with 100 to 150 ml of dilute methylene blue solution or sterile milk. This step also rules out the possibility of another unrecognized bladder laceration. The milk is preferred by some, as it does not

identified at laparotomy. If an intestinal injury has occurred and multiple adhesions remain, it may be much more practical to proceed directly to a laparotomy.

Ureteral Injury

Injury to the ureter during vaginal hysterectomy is uncommon. Ureteral injury is asymptomatic in many patients, and therefore is probably underrecognized and underreported. Ureteral injury is less common with vaginal hysterectomy than with abdominal hysterectomy—probably a phenomenon of case selection more than anything else. Ureteral injury is more likely to occur during vaginal hysterectomy for severe prolapse, anterior colporrhaphy, or culdoplasty.

In 1962 Hofmeister and Wolfgram described the relation between vaginal hysterectomy ligatures and the ureters.[8] They obtained preoperative and postoperative intravenous pyelograms on 114 patients undergoing vaginal hysterectomy and found no instance of postoperative ureteral injury. They further studied the problem first by placing radiopaque ureteral catheters and wire sutures and then measuring the distance between the wire sutures and the ureters at various points on multiple radiographs obtained during the procedure. Later, they took these measurements from the applied Heaney clamps under fluoroscopy. The distance from the clamps to the ureters in the paracervical tissue varied from 2 to 3 cm. Clamps applied adjacent to the cervix at the level of the uterine arteries measured 3 cm from the ureters. It was also noted that anterior retraction under the bladder lifted the ureters as much as 1 cm away from the zone of danger. When transfixation sutures of the paracervical tissues were attached to the corners of the vagina, the distance of the closest wire suture was measured at 1.5 cm from the ureter. When a Heaney clamp was placed on the infundibulopelvic ligament, the fluoroscopically measured distance to the ureter was 1 cm. Cruikshank and Kovac have utilized preoperative computed tomography (CT) scans and intraoperative ureteral dissection to evaluate the anatomic changes of the ureter during vaginal hysterectomy, especially as related to the uterosacral–cardinal ligament complex.[3]

The results of these studies reinforce our knowledge of the proper surgical techniques needed to avoid injury to the ureter: proper traction on the cervix and retraction of the bladder, proper placement of the clamps, and care in the manner in which hemostasis is obtained when it is necessary. Ureteral injury is unlikely to be recognized as an intraoperative complication. However, when this possibility is suspected, such as in the patient who has required additional suturing of the parametrial tissues for hemostasis, the status of the ureters can be evaluated as described above by the cystoscopic observation of indigo carmine exiting from the ureteral orifices or with retrograde ureterography. An intravenous pyelogram may also be performed intraoperatively.

If it appears that a mild ureteral injury has occurred (i.e., inclusion in a large pedicle) and a stent can be passed, the injury may be managed conservatively. Otherwise a laparotomy with prompt correction of the problem is the best course of action. At laparotomy the space of Retzius is opened, and the anterior fundus of the bladder is opened vertically. An attempt is made to pass a ureteral catheter up the ureteral orifice. The catheter may be stopped promptly by a ligature or may be seen to exit from a transected portion of the ureter. In either case use of the catheter helps identify the site of injury. If the ureteral catheter passes with difficulty, the ureter is probably kinked by a suture, which should be identified if possible and removed. If the catheter does not pass, the ureter above it is mobilized and dissected down to the point of injury. In some cases the ureter can be unobstructed by simply removing a ligating suture. A ureteral stent and pelvic drain should be left in place so long as the injury to the ureter itself does not appear significant.

If there seems to be significant injury or transection of the ureter, ureteroneocystotomy is then necessary. The uninjured portion of the ureter is mobilized and transected above the injury. A site is chosen toward the posterior aspect of the bladder fundus for the ureteral implantation. A tonsil clamp is placed through the bladder outward, and the ureter is pulled through this opening, which should not be tight. The ureteral orifice is splayed, and the full thickness of the ureter is sutured to the bladder mucosa and muscularis with approximating 4-0 chromic catgut sutures. The ureter can readily be brought under a small submucosal tunnel prior to making the anastomosis if desired. A double-J ureteral stent is left in place, and a closed-suction drain is used in the pelvis near the anastomosis. A 20 French suprapubic catheter is placed, and the bladder is closed in layers as previously described with a running stitch of 3-0 chromic suture. The integrity of the repair should be gently tested while simultaneously observing for reflux from the distal portion of the transected ureter. A 20 French transurethral Foley catheter is also placed. Bladder drainage should be maintained for 7 to 10 days, although one of these catheters can be removed when there is no more gross hematuria. The patient is likely to experience bladder spasms, which can be treated with antispasmodic agents. The ureteral catheter can be removed in approximately 4 weeks, and an intravenous pyelogram is obtained shortly thereafter.

Hemorrhage

The final intraoperative complication to be discussed is hemorrhage, which generally stems from uterine or ovarian vessels. As with the other complications, prevention is best accomplished using careful surgical technique. Hemorrhage can be prevented with controlled sharp dissection within the proper tissue planes, secure ligation of pedicles without intervening gaps, careful placement of clamps, avoidance of traction on vascular pedicles, and the use of secure clamps that do not allow tissue slippage.

The area of greatest risk is the infundibulopelvic ligament. In the event that this pedicle is lost or incompletely tied, immediate laparotomy may be required. As one attempts to retrieve this pedicle the ureter potentially becomes endangered. Proper selection of cases for transvaginal salpingo-oophorectomy is probably the single most important step for preventing this problem. Transvaginal management of the adnexa was discussed at length in Chapter 3.

It must be kept in mind that there is less control over back-bleeding during vaginal hysterectomy than during abdominal hysterectomy. Such bleeding is sometimes brisk and is best controlled by promptly completing the hysterectomy. If the paracervical pedicles are lost through suture breakage, slippage from the clamp, or some other reason, it is usually not difficult to retrieve these tissues for reclamping and suturing. The cut edge of the pedicle should be grasped with long Allis clamps (Fig. 4-4) followed either by directly suturing the pedicle or first placing a right-angle clamp (Fig. 4-5) and then suturing the pedicle. Additional small areas of bleeding around or between the pedicles can often be managed with the careful application of cautery. If the uterine pedicle should escape, the uterine arteries do not retract, and retrieval is generally feasible. As with the paracervical tissues, care must be taken when reclamping and resuturing this pedicle not to incorporate tissues more lateral than those originally intended, as this may injure the ureter.

After ligation of the uterine pedicle, traction on the uterus occasionally causes a tear in the broad ligament above it. This problem can often be avoided by incorporating the anterior and posterior uterine serosa in the uterine pedicle clamp. If a tear should occur, however, it generally does not result in significant hemorrhage. Proceeding with ligation of the utero-ovarian pedicle usually secures hemostasis. With good exposure, any small bleeders from the upper broad ligament may be cauterized or ligated. If the utero-ovarian pedicle should be lost, it can also generally be readily retrieved and resutured. The ureter is distant from this pedicle and is not in danger of injury. A common problem with this pedicle is bleeding from the fallopian tube or ovary as a result of inadvertent trauma to these structures. Bleeding from the fallopian tube can be

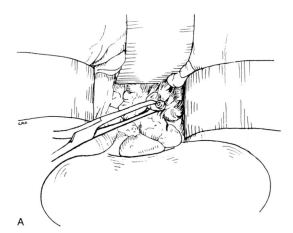

Figure 4-4. (A & B) Bleeding site is grasped with a long Allis clamp. Gentle traction is then applied to distance this tissue from the ureter.

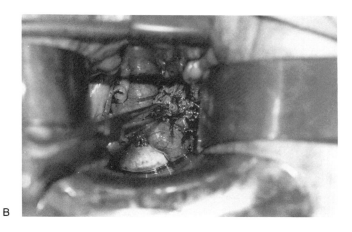

controlled by pressure, ligature, or the careful application of cautery. Bleeding from a traumatized ovary, especially in the presence of a functional cyst, is more difficult to stop. Cautery is frequently unsuccessful and often exacerbates the problem. Suturing may also worsen the problem and further predisposes the patient to a postoperative ovarian abscess. The bleeding frequently stops with simple observation or pressure. Otherwise a transvaginal ovarian cystectomy or oophorectomy may be necessary.

A lost infundibulopelvic ligament pedicle is the most difficult and dangerous to retrieve. With careful placement of retractors and good lighting, however, the pedicle can usually be visualized and grasped transvaginally with a long Allis clamp. A long right-angle clamp may then be carefully placed just above the Allis clamp. The proximity of the ureter must be kept in mind as the clamp is placed. If it is apparent that bleeding during or immediately after completion of the vaginal hysterectomy cannot readily be controllable transvaginally, a laparotomy should be promptly performed.

Figure 4-5. (A & B) Right-angle clamp is placed across bleeding tissue held by the Allis clamp. Using this narrower clamp rather than another pedicle clamp helps to maintain a safe distance from the ureter.

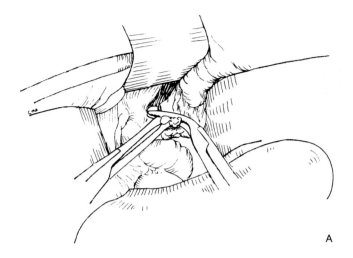

A

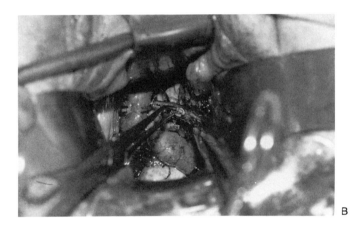

B

Needless to say, there must be close communication between the gynecologic surgeon, the anesthesiologist, and the remainder of the operating room staff in order to maintain optimum organization and expedition of the patient's care. The anesthesiologist must be given an accurate understanding of what is transpiring so he or she can maintain the patient's intravascular volume, hemoglobin, and coagulating ability.

At laparotomy bleeding sites are identified and hemostasis is obtained with metal clips, cautery, or carefully placed sutures. Full knowledge of the location of the ureters is important during these maneuvers. If extensive blood loss has occurred, the surgeon should keep in mind the possibility of a dilutional coagulopathy. It is sometimes appropriate to tightly pack the pelvis while waiting for replenishment of blood volume, platelets, and other coagulation factors. In some situations it is difficult to identify and obtain hemostasis of individual bleeding vessels, in which case it may be helpful to ligate the anterior division of both internal iliac arteries.

References

1. Browne DS, Frazer MI. Hysterectomy revisited. Aust NZ J Obstet Gynaecol 31:148–152, 1991
2. Copenhaver EH. Vaginal hysterectomy: an analysis of indication and complications among 1,000 operations. Am J Obstet Gynecol 84:123–128, 1962
3. Cruikshank SH, Kovac SR. Anatomic changes of ureter during vaginal hysterectomy. Contemp Obstet Gynecol February:38–53, 1993
4. Dicker RC, Greenspan JR, Strauss LT, et al. Complications of abdominal and vaginal hysterectomy among women of reproductive age in the United States: the collaborative review of sterilization. Am J Obstet Gynecol 144:841–848, 1982
5. Falk HC, Bunkin IA. A study of 500 vaginal hysterectomies. Am J Obstet Gynecol 52:623–630, 1946
6. Gitsch G, Berger E, Tatra G. Trends in thirty years of vaginal hysterectomy. Surg Gynecol Obstet 172:207–210, 1991
7. Gray LA. Indications, techniques, and complications in vaginal hysterectomy. Obstet Gynecol 28:714–722, 1966
8. Hofmeister FJ, Wolfgram RL. Methods of demonstrating measurement relationships between vaginal hysterectomy ligatures and the ureters. Am J Obstet Gynecol 83:938–948, 1962
9. Ledger WJ, Campbell C, Wilson JR. Postoperative adnexal infections. Obstet Gynecol 31:83–89, 1968
10. Livengood CH III, Addison WA. Adnexal abscess as a delayed complication of vaginal hysterectomy. Am J Obstet Gynecol 143:596–597, 1982
11. Perineau M, Monrozies X, Reme JM. Complications of hysterectomy. Rev Fr Gynecol Obstet 87:120–125, 1992
12. Pratt JH, Daikoku NH. Obesity and vaginal hysterectomy. J Reprod Med 35:945–949, 1990
13. Pratt JH, Galloway JR. Vaginal hysterectomy in patients less than 36 or more than 60 years of age. Am J Obstet Gynecol 84:123–128, 1962
14. Rosenzweig BA, Seifer DB, Grant WD, et al. Urologic injury during vaginal hysterectomy: a case-control study. J Gynecol Surg 6:27–32, 1990
15. Stanhope CR, Wilson TO, Utz WJ, Smith LH, O'Brien PC. Suture entrapment and secondary ureteral obstruction. Am J Obstet Gynecol 164:1513–1519, 1991

Suggested Reading

Heaney NS. A report of 565 vaginal hysterectomies performed for benign pelvic disease. Am J Obstet Gynecol 28:751–755, 1934

Kudo R, Yamauchi O, Okazaki T, et al. Vaginal hysterectomy without ligation of the ligaments of the cervix uteri. Surg Obstet Gynecol 170:299–305, 1990

Leventhal ML, Lazarus ML. Total abdominal and vaginal hysterectomy, a comparison. Am J Obstet Gynecol 61:289–299, 1951

Pratt JH. Operative and postoperative difficulties of vaginal hysterectomy. Obstet Gynecol 21:220–226, 1963

Tancer ML. Observations on prevention and management of vesicovaginal fistula after total hysterectomy. Surg Gynecol Obstet 175:501–506, 1992

Tasche LW. 1700 Vaginal hysterectomies in a general surgical practice. Minn Med 51:1705–1711, 1968.

White SC, Watel LJ, Wade ME. Comparison of abdominal and vaginal hysterectomies: a review of 600 operations. Obstet Gynecol 37:530–537, 1971

Wilson JR, Black JR. Ovarian abscess. Am J Obstet Gynecol 90:34–43, 1964

5

Enlarged Uterus

*In general, the capable surgeon selects the vaginal route for hysterectomy based
on a number of anatomic factors, including a relatively normal size uterus.
When feasible, the operation, successfully completed through the vagina, affords
the patient a quick and easy recovery. With little if any additional morbidity,
certain uteri that are moderately enlarged can also be readily removed transvaginally while retaining the advantages of the vaginal approach. This chapter
describes selection factors and operative techniques for the transvaginal removal
of enlarged uteri. A versatile surgeon, who can adapt his or her technique to
each individual case, becomes an even more important element to the successful
transvaginal removal of enlarged uteri. The more difficult cases require an experienced surgeon using good surgical judgment.*

The removal of enlarged uteri transvaginally is a concept that dates
back at least 100 years. Before the turn of the century, when laparotomy was relatively unsafe, this operation was especially relevant.
The summarized history of vaginal hysterectomy by Gray in 1955
contains many references to the transvaginal morcellation of enlarged uteri during the nineteenth century.[2] Today laparotomy is
safe in most patients, which leads the gynecologic surgeon to ques-
tion the logic behind struggling to remove an enlarged uterus
through the vagina. The reduced morbidity associated with vaginal
hysterectomy compared with abdominal hysterectomy was dis-

cussed in earlier chapters. Based on a review of retrospective studies of patients who had undergone vaginal hysterectomy with and without morcellation, it appears that little if any additional morbidity is incurred when morcellation is necessary to complete the hysterectomy.

In a retrospective study Kovac compared patients who had undergone vaginal hysterectomy, vaginal hysterectomy with morcellation, and abdominal hysterectomy.[4] His results also showed no additional morbidity with transvaginal morcellation and, along with the other studies, support the idea that vaginal hysterectomy with or without morcellation in properly selected patients creates less morbidity than abdominal hysterectomy. Depending on the size of the pelvis and the configuration of the uterus, transvaginal removal of the intact uterus is generally not possible for uteri that are 10 to 12 weeks (gestational) size or larger. Segmental or piecemeal removal of the uterus is necessary if such hysterectomies are to be completed transvaginally. "Uterine morcellation" may also facilitate transvaginal hysterectomy when the pelvis is relatively small or there is a relative lack of uterine descent. This chapter deals with various techniques of morcellation that facilitate transvaginal removal of an enlarged uterus.

The reported frequency of morcellation performed with vaginal hysterectomy varies from 0% to 76%. This wide range probably relates to the varied experience and philosophies of the gynecologic surgeons.

Patient Selection

Proper patient selection is the key to successful removal of enlarged uteri transvaginally. This is done by a careful pelvic examination, frequently with the final decision made during the examination under anesthesia. The anatomic factors discussed in Chapter 2 are perhaps more important when contemplating transvaginal removal of an enlarged uterus.

With experience, the gynecologic surgeon gains a sense of which enlarged uteri can be removed through the vagina. Despite its size the uterus must be clearly mobile. Mobility of the enlarged fundal portion of the uterus is best determined during a bimanual pelvic examination and the mobility of the lower uterine segment by applying a tenaculum to the cervix and moving the cervix up into the pelvis and out again. This is also the time to determine surgical accessibility to the lower uterine segment, which is prerequisite for safe conduct of the transvaginal approach. It should be apparent to the gynecologic surgeon that the surgery can readily proceed to the level of the uterine artery pedicles before any type of morcellation is necessary. Mobility and descensus of the lower uterine segment must be present. The gynecologic surgeon must be wary of the elongated cervix, which can make surgical access to the lower uterine segment appear a good deal easier than it actually is. Leiomyomas of the cervix or lower uterine segment may interfere substantially with safe ligation of the lower pedicles, especially when the myomas are subvesicle or intraligamentous. If there appears to be good surgical access to the lower uterine segment and good mobility of the uterine fundus, it is likely that transvaginal removal of the uterus can be completed successfully. The size and configuration of the uterine fundus are two other important factors that must be carefully evaluated when deciding on the best approach. Diffuse uterine enlargement into a markedly "plump" uterus and the presence of anterior or lateral myomas tend to make transvaginal removal more difficult. A uterine fundus containing multiple discrete or predominantly posterior fundal myomas lends itself to transvaginal removal. With such favorable configurations, even large uteri can be delivered transvaginally.

There are no strict guidelines regarding uterine size, and each case must be approached individually based on the gynecologic surgeon's best judgment. Pratt and Gunnlaugsson in 1970 reported that 14 of 109 morcellated uteri weighed in excess of 300 g, with the largest being 700 g.[6] Kovac in 1986 reported a mean weight of 163 g for 554 morcellated uteri, with a range of 100 to 750 g.[4] Grody in 1989 reported the successful transvaginal removal of 320 of 324 consecutive myomatous uteri weighing between 190 and 810 g.[3] In 1990 Kudo et al. reported a uterine weight in excess of 500 g for 1213 of 9230 vaginal hysterectomies; in fact, 108 of the uteri were in excess of 1000 g.[5] These results are interesting and indicate that even large uteri can be removed transvaginally in a reasonable manner. The importance of the expertise of the surgeons who published these results cannot be overemphasized.

As experience and manual dexterity are gained, the gynecologic surgeon becomes increasingly adept at removing larger uteri transvaginally. For most gynecologic surgeons it is probably reasonable to approach selected uteri up to 12 to 14 weeks' (gestational) size transvaginally. Because of the bulk alone and the relative immobility of a bulky fundus, transvaginal removal of large uteri becomes an increasingly difficult struggle, with prolonged operative time and increased blood loss. Although again a matter of individual judgment for each case, uteri larger than 12 to 14 weeks' (gestational) size are generally removed much more readily transabdominally.

For certain patients, such as those who are obese, those with chronic severe respiratory disease, or other medically compromised women, it may be worthwhile to struggle a bit to remove selected, somewhat larger uteri transvaginally. Although not ideal, little is

Figure 5-1. Useful instruments for transvaginal morcellation of the enlarged uterus. *Left to right:* three triple-tooth tenaculums, extra long and heavy scissors, single-tooth tenaculums (*top*), towel clamps (*bottom*), Bovie with extender.

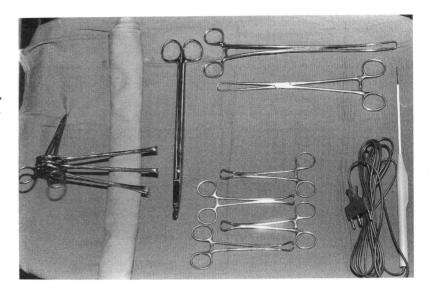

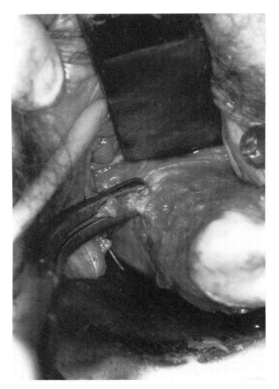

Figure 5-2. Uterine artery pedicle is clamped. In general, vaginal hysterectomy should proceed at least to the ligation of this pedicle before beginning morcellation.

lost if it is realized without undue delay that the hysterectomy would be better completed transabdominally.

Preparation

Most uteri considered for transvaginal morcellation are enlarged owing to leiomyomas, although in some cases the enlargement is the result of diffuse adenomyosis. When contemplating transvaginal morcellation of the uterus the surgeon must be confident that no uterine malignancy is present.

The patient who is to undergo transvaginal removal of an enlarged uterus should be typed and cross-matched for possible blood transfusion and be scheduled for a longer than usual operative time. Expert assistance is necessary, and a number of additional instruments may be useful (Fig. 5-1).

Initial Steps

Transvaginal removal of the enlarged uterus proceeds in a routine fashion to the uterine artery pedicles (Fig. 5-2). The nature of the pelvic mass should be confirmed through the posterior colpotomy

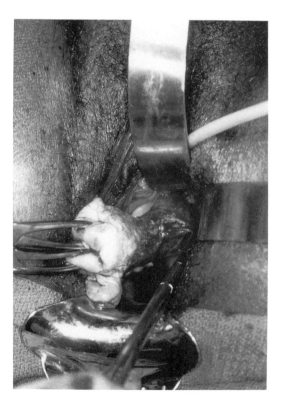

Figure 5-3. Portion of the broad ligament is clamped just above the uterine artery. When feasible, it is helpful to ligate this pedicle before beginning morcellation. It is probably best not to go higher, however, as it would risk avulsion of the remaining attachments when strong traction is placed on the uterus during morcellation and delivery.

TABLE 5-1. Methods of reducing uterine size for vaginal hysterectomy on the enlarged uterus

Surgical methods
Myomectomy
Posterior fundal morcellation
Hemisection ± morcellation
Intramyometrial coring
Medical method
GnRH analogues

incision. If an additional pedicle on the broad ligament can be ligated prior to beginning morcellation, it should be done (Fig. 5-3). If the uterine fundus cannot be delivered through the posterior colpotomy but it still appears reasonable to proceed transvaginally, several options exist. These various surgical options are designed to reduce the internal pelvic volume of the uterine fundus to a critical point that allows it to be delivered through the vaginal cuff (Fig. 5-4). The techniques that can be used to accomplish this step are not mutually exclusive and frequently are combined in order to proceed in the most advantageous manner apparent to each case. Versatility in the application of the various morcellation techniques is a key factor to successful transvaginal removal of enlarged uteri.

The most common or best described techniques used to accomplish delivery of the enlarged uterine fundus are listed in Table 5-1;

Figure 5-4. Large uterus is morcellated to the point that transvaginal delivery is possible.

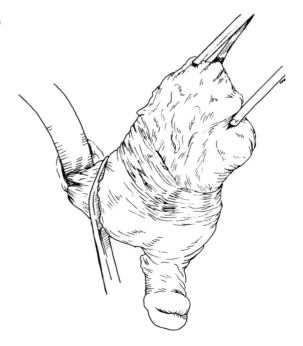

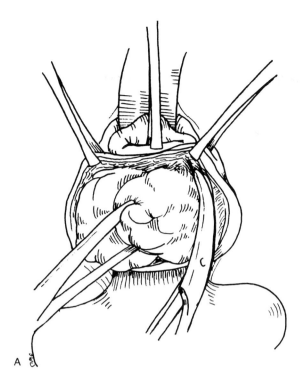

Figure 5-5. (A) Transvaginal myomectomy. (B) Readily accessible midline leiomyoma. (C) Transvaginal delivery of a large myoma.

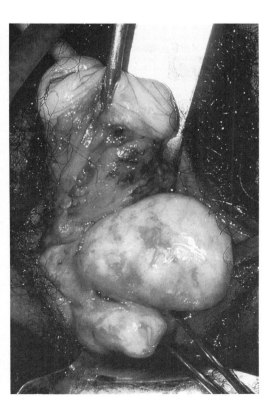

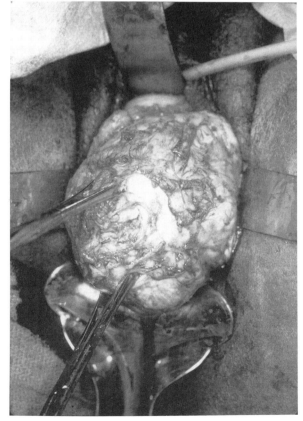

Figure 5-6. Excision of the exocervix with the distal endocervical canal in order to reduce bacterial contamination of the peritoneal cavity during uterine manipulation.

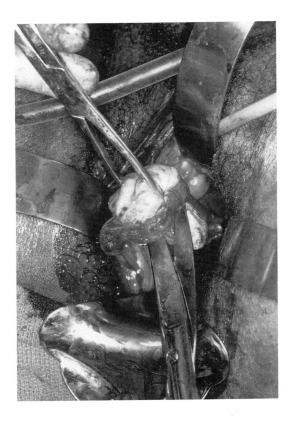

they include myomectomy, posterior fundal morcellation, uterine hemisection with or without morcellation, and intramyometrial coring.

Myomectomy, frequently carried out during the course of such hysterectomies, can be done easily; and when the surgeon stays within the capsule it is safe and generally fairly bloodless (Fig. 5-5). Removal of myomas reduces the uterine size and often provides better exposure.

Cervicectomy is sometimes used adjunctively with these techniques to reduce bacterial contamination of the operative site and to facilitate "flipping" of the uterine fundus (Fig. 5-6). These potential advantages must be balanced in some cases against the usefulness of the cervix for traction or orientation.

Posterior Fundal Morcellation

Beginning at the lower posterior fundus, morcellation successively removes quadrangular pieces, working cephalad until the fundus can be delivered (Fig. 5-7). Tenaculums are "walked" up the posterior fundus, delivering whatever portion of the fundus that can be readily retrieved into the operative field. It must be possible to pull

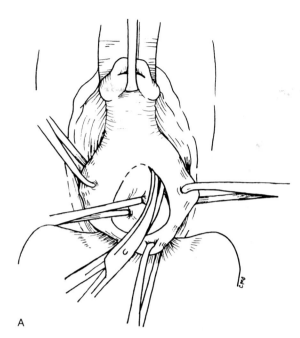

Figure 5-7. (A) Posterior fundal morcellation. (B) Posterior uterine fundus is partially morcellated and delivered. (C) Portion of posterior uterine fundus being excised.

Continued on next page.

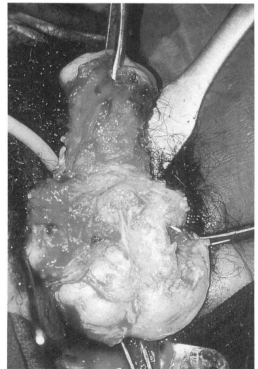

B

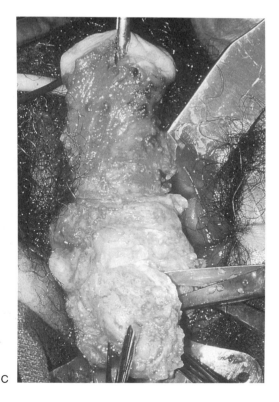

C

Figure 5-7 *Continued*
(D) Following excision,
further delivery of the uterine
fundus is possible
(E) Morcellated uterus.

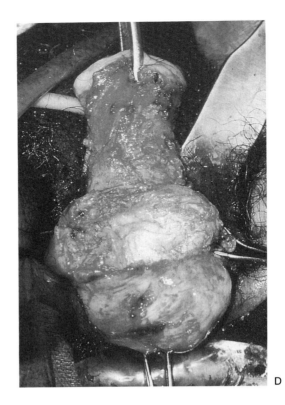

D

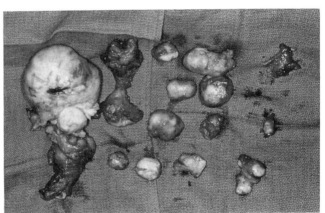

E

a reasonable portion of the posterior uterine fundus into the operative field if this technique is to be used. Additional tenaculums are placed laterally to maintain control within the bounds of the broad ligaments and yet allow maximum feasible removal. Control of the morcellation process is thus maintained by one superior and two lateral tenaculums. A tenaculum applied to the piece of tissue to be excised is also helpful for the purpose of traction. Continuous traction on these tenaculums also reduces bleeding during the mor-

cellation process. Care must be taken not extend the resection laterally into the broad ligaments or through the anterior surface of the
uterus, as the latter may cause injury or produce marked distortion,
leading to disorientation of the remaining uterus.

During the posterior fundal morcellation process, it is efficacious
to perform myomectomies as the myomas are encountered. If it is
apparent that more tissue can be removed from areas of previous
quadrangular excision, it should be done as necessary to accomplish fundal delivery. Occasionally posterior fundal morcellation is
exhausted, and the fundus still cannot be delivered, or access to
the adnexal pedicles is not adequate. Hemisection of the remainder
of the uterus with or without further morcellation is an excellent
method to finally achieve delivery of the uterine fundus in such in-
stances.

Uterine Hemisection

Uterine hemisection with or without morcellation is another common method for delivering an enlarged uterine fundus. Hemisection
of a mild to moderately enlarged uterus, thereby reducing the
mass by one-half, may be all that is needed to accomplish delivery
of the fundus through the vaginal cuff (Fig. 5-8).

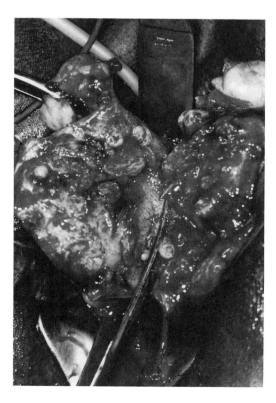

Figure 5-8. Moderately
enlarged myomatous uterus is
being hemisected to facilitate
vaginal delivery and accession
to the upper attachments.
Note the cephalad protection
afforded by the Heaney
retractor.

Hemisection may begin at the cervix or the fundus. Using tenaculums and a finger or heavy instrument such as a malleable ribbon behind the uterus for protection and guidance, the uterine fundus is completely divided. If the uterus is too large or too inaccessible to be completely divided or if neither half can be delivered after division, some additional morcellation becomes necessary. As hemisection proceeds superiorly, tenaculums are applied and successive tri-

Figure 5-9. (A & B) Uterine hemisection with morcellation.

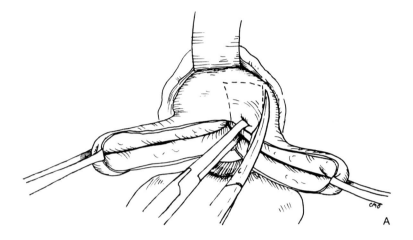

A

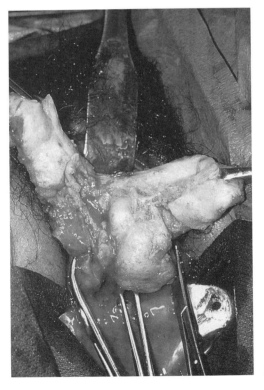

B

angular or quadrangular pieces are excised (Fig. 5-9). This process may, of course, include multiple myomectomies. Again, continuous downward traction on the fundus reduces bleeding. Excisions are carried out from both sides of the hemisection incision and separately from the anterior and posterior uterine fundus until the hemisection can be completed or the fundus delivered. When excising the tissue, care again must be taken not to extend into the broad ligaments.

Intramyometrial Coring

Another technique for transvaginal delivery of an enlarged uterine fundus is intramyometrial coring. This technique is well suited for removal of a diffusely enlarged uterine fundus, the lower portion of which descends well and is thus accessible to the surgeon. This method is technically somewhat more difficult than the other methods of fundal reduction, especially with large uteri. With experience, however, it is effective; and a large series has been reported using this method with good results.[4]

One of the proposed advantages of intramyometrial coring is avoidance of the endometrial cavity, although such avoidance is frequently not possible. In addition, it is not clear that any significant harm results from entering the endometrial cavity during morcellation. Other proposed advantages include a safer transvaginal ap-

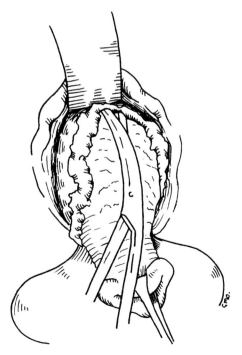

Figure 5-10. Intramyometrial coring.

Figure 5-11. (A) Gradual delivery of the cored portion of the uterus. (B–C) Intra-myometrial coring is done to a "critical" point of the upper uterine fundus, after which the entire mass can be delivered. The utero-ovarian pedicle is then clamped as usual.

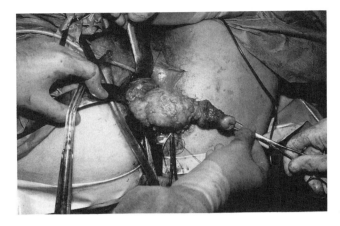

A

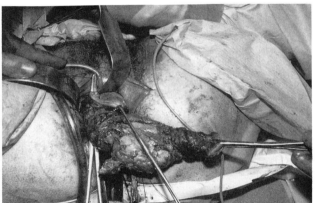

B

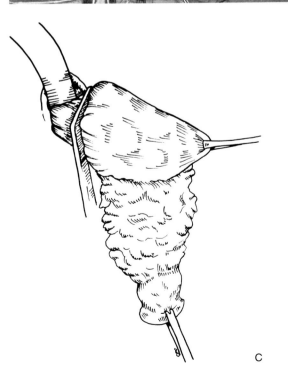

C

proach in the presence of intraligamentous or subvesicle leiomyo-
mata and avoidance of adhesions until they can be brought into
the clear view of the surgeon.

Intramyometrial coring generally begins with a circumferential incision into the lower fundus near the point where it begins to ex-
pand. Large, heavy Mayo scissors are well suited for this purpose.
The incision is continued circumferentially and cephalad through
the myometrium while constant traction is applied to the cervix
(Fig. 5-10). Gradual delivery of the cored portion should be noted
(Fig. 5-11a). Good exposure given by capable assistants is important. The direction of the dissection parallels the uterine serosa. A
shell of myometrium is left that is thick enough to avoid perfora-
tion through the serosa or tearing of the remaining shell. Ideally,
entry into the endometrial cavity is also avoided.

The difficult aspect of the technique is carrying out a path of dissection that ultimately achieves delivery of the fundus. If the uterus
is not more than 10 to 12 weeks' (gestational) size, a line of dissection through the middle of the myometrium should work well. A
common error is to dissect a small core that is inadequate to reduce
the volume sufficiently to effect delivery of the fundus. Especially
when dealing with a large uterus, it is generally more effective to
keep the dissection close to the uterine serosa. The large core can
be secondarily partially morcellated as needed during dissection. As
with the other techniques, multiple myomectomies are frequently
performed in the process. The volume of the uterus is eventually
critically reduced, which allows its delivery as well as ligation of
the adnexal pedicles (Fig. 5-11b,c). As intramyometrial coring proceeds, it may be apparent at some point that an alternative technique would complete delivery of the fundus more efficaciously.

Management of the Adnexae

After removal of the uterus the adnexae are evaluated (Fig. 5-12).
Feasibility of transvaginal adnexectomy in such patients can be assessed only at this time.

Gonadotropin-Releasing Hormone Agonist

A relatively new preoperative medical management may reduce the
need for extensive morcellation. The treatment is to administer
a gonadotropin releasing hormone agonist (GnRH-a), which by
down-regulating the pituitary gonadotropin cell receptors produces
temporary medical castration. This therapy can reduce the uterine
myoma mass by about 50% in 3 months. This smaller uterus may
then be more easily removed vaginally.

Figure 5-12. Enlarged and partially morcellated uterus is delivered and the utero-ovarian pedicle clamped. The right adnexa is now accessible for removal.

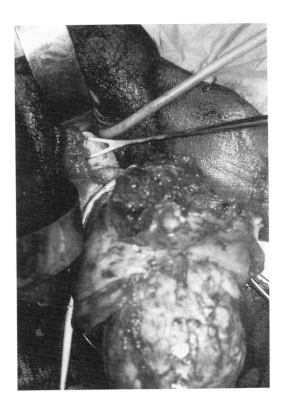

Summary

As experience and dexterity are gained, the gynecologic surgeon develops a sense, during examination, of which enlarged uteri can be reasonably removed transvaginally. An individualized approach and a versatile surgical armamentarium are the important elements to safely and effectively removing large uteri transvaginally.

References

1. Dicker RC, Greenspan JR, Strauss LT, et al. Complications of abdominal and vaginal hysterectomy among women of reproductive age in the United States: the collaborative review of sterilization. Am J Obstet Gynecol 144:841–848, 1982
2. Gray LA. Vaginal hysterectomy. Charles C Thomas. Springfield, IL, 1955
3. Grody MHT. Vaginal hysterectomy: the large uterus. J Gynecol Surg 5:301–312, 1989
4. Kovac SR. Intramyometrial coring as an adjunct to vaginal hysterectomy. Obstet Gynecol 67:131–136, 1986
5. Kudo R, Yamauchi O, Okazaki T, et al. Vaginal hysterectomy without ligation of the ligaments of the cervix uteri. Surg Gynecol Obstet 170:299–305, 1990

6. Pratt JH, Gunnlaugsson GH. Vaginal hysterectomy by morcellation. Mayo Clin Proc 45:374–387, 1970

Suggested Reading

Allen E, Peterson LF. Versatility of vaginal hysterectomy technique. Obstet Gynecol 3:240–247, 1954

Bradford WZ, Bradford WB, Woltz JHE, Brown CW. Experiences with vaginal hysterectomy. Am J Obstet Gynecol 68:540–548, 1954

Campbell ZB. A report on 2,798 vaginal hysterectomies. Am J Obstet Gynecol 52:598–613, 1946

Copenhaver EH. Vaginal hysterectomy: an analysis of indication and complications among 1,000 operations. Am J Obstet Gynecol 84:123–128, 1962

Easterday CL, Grimes DA, Riggs JA. Hysterectomy in the United States. Obstet Gynecol 62:203–212, 1983

Falk HC, Bunkin IA. A study of 500 vaginal hysterectomies. Am J Obstet Gynecol 52:623–630, 1946

Falk HC, Soichet S. The technique of vaginal hysterectomy. Clin Obstet Gynecol 15:703–754, 1972

Garceau E. Vaginal hysterectomy as done in France. Am J Obstet Gynecol 31:305–346, 1895

Harris BA. Vaginal hysterectomy in a community hospital. NY State J Med 76:1304–1307, 1976

Heaney NS. A report of 565 vaginal hysterectomies performed for benign pelvic disease. Am J Obstet Gynecol 28:751–755, 1934

Hoffman MS, DeCesare S, Kalter C. Abdominal hysterectomy versus transvaginal morcellation for the removal of enarged uteri. Am J Obstet Gynecol (In Press, 1994)

Ingram JM, Withers RW, Wright HL. The debated indications for vaginal hysterectomy. South Med J 51:869–872, 1958

Lash AF. A method for reducing the size of the uterus in vaginal hysterectomy. Am J Obstet Gynecol 42:452–459, 1941

Leventhal ML, Lazarus ML. Total abdominal and vaginal hysterectomy, a comparison. Am J Obstet Gynecol 61:289–299, 1951

Porges RF. Changing indications for vaginal hysterectomy. Am J Obstet Gynecol 136:153–158, 1980

Schneider D, Golan A, Bukousky I, Pansky M, Caspi E. GNRH analogue-induced uterine shrinkage enabling a vaginal hysterectomy and repair in large leiomyomatous uteri. Obstet Gynecol 78:540–541, 1991

Stovall TG, Ling FW, Henry LC, Woodruff MR. A randomized trial evaluating leuprolide acetate before hysterectomy as treatment for leiomyomas. Am J Obstet Gynecol 164:1420–1425, 1991

6

Lack of Descensus

Methods for overcoming the obstacle of uterine enlargement when performing a vaginal hysterectomy were discussed in Chapter 5. Another significant obstacle to the vaginal approach is a significant lack of uterine descensus. Many other anatomic factors play an important role in the feasibility of vaginal hysterectomy. With experience and good judgment, the surgeon is usually able to select patients for vaginal hysterectomy in whom a relative lack of descensus can be readily overcome. Some operative techniques are described that help the surgeon obtain access to the more superiorly placed pedicles encountered with these uteri. Access to the ovarian pedicles is not necessarily as difficult, and they should be approached on an individual basis as is discussed.

One of the most widely accepted criteria for vaginal hysterectomy has been pelvic relaxation with descensus or prolapse. The term uterine descensus is ambiguous but is generally used to imply that traction on a cervix of normal length can bring it close to the introitus or beyond. Uterine prolapse has frequently been defined in terms of three degrees of severity, although these definitions have not been uniform (Table 6-1). Throughout the history of vaginal hysterectomy, its most common indication has been uterine prolapse or pelvic relaxation. Many of the currently accepted indications for hysterectomy, however, such as cervical intraepithelial neoplasia III, persistent abnormal bleeding, and leiomyomas, do

TABLE 6-1. Definitions of uterine prolapse

First degree	Second degree	Third degree (total, procidentia)	Source
Descent that does not involve protrusion of cervix at introitus	Cervix protrudes	Entire uterus pushed outside introitus	a
Cervix comes to introitus	Cervix is well outside of vagina	Entire uterus external	b
Some descent of uterus; cervix has not reached introitus	Cervix alone or with part of uterus passes through introitus	Protrusion of entire uterus beyond introitus	c
Cervix almost reaches introitus	Cervix visible at introitus	Cervix protudes beyond introitus	d
Not given	With straining, cervix reaches hymeneal ring	With straining, cervix reaches beyond introitus Complete: entire vaginal canal inverted	e
Cervix descends to introitus	Descent of uterus through intoritus	Uterus prolapsed out of vagina	f
Cervix descends to introitus	Cervix protrudes through introitus	Entire uterus protrudes through vaginal outlet	g
Uterine descent within vagina	Uterine descent beyond intoritus	Complete eversion of vagina; uterus usually lies below introitus unless marked cervical elongation	h
Prolapse into upper barrel of vagina	Prolapse to the introitus	Cervix and uterus prolapse out through the introitus	i
Incomplete: uterus descends only partly down vagina	Moderate: uterus descends to introitus, and cervix protrudes slightly beyond	Entire cervix and uterus protrude beynd introitus; vagina inverted	j
Uterus has descended only a slight distance into vagina	Cervix appears outside vulva	Uterus protrudes through introitus	k
Uterus descends, cervix remains within vagina	Cervix appears partially or totally outside the vaginal orifice	Entire uterus outside the vaginal orifice	l
Cervix lies between ischial spines and introitus	Cervix protrudes thorugh introitus	Both cervix and body of uterus passed through introitus; vagina inverted	m

a Netter F. Reproductive System. Ciba, 1977. Rochester, p. 146.
b Rommey SL, Gray MJ, Little AB, et al. Gynecology and Obstetrics: The Health Care of Women, 1981. McGraw-Hill Book Co., New York, p. 969.
c Danforth DN, Scott JR. Obstetrics and Gynecology, 1986. (5th ed) JB Lippincott Co., Philadelphia, p. 964.
d Rosenwaks Z, Benjamin F, Stone ML. Gynecology: Principles and Practice, 1987. Macmillan Publishing Co., New York, p. 490.
e Jones HW III, Wentz AC, Burnett LS. Novak's Textbook of Gynecology, 1988. (11th ed) Williams & Wilkins, Baltimore, pp. 456–457.
f Dunnihoo DR. Fundamentals of Gynecology and Obstetrics, 1990. JB Lippincott Co., Philadelphia, p. 57.
g Clarke-Pearson DL, Dawood MY. Green's Gynecology: Essentials of Clinical Practice, 1990. (4th ed) Little, Brown and Co., Boston, p. 398.
h Mackey EV, Beischer NA, Cox LW, Wood C. Illustrated Textbook of Gynecology, 1983. WB Saunders Co., Philadelphia, p. 299.
i Herbst AL, Mishell DR, Jr, Stenchever MA, Droegmueller W. Comprehensive Gynecology, 1992. Mosby Year Book, St. Louis, p. 591.
j Pernoll ML, Benson RC. Current Obstetric and Gynecologic Diagnosis and Treatment, 1987. (6th ed) Appleton & Large, Norwalk, p. 760.
k Barber HRK, Fields DH, Kaufman SA. Quick Reference to Ob-Gyn Procedures, 1990. (3rd ed) JB Lippincott Co., Philadelphia, pp. 356–57.
l Wynn RM. Obstetrics and Gynecology: The Clinical Core, 1988. (4th ed) Lea & Febiger, Philadelphia, p. 220.
m Wilson JR, Carrington ER, Ledger WJ, Laros RK, Jr, Mattox JH. Obstetrics and Gynecology, 1987. (8th ed) The C.V. Mosby Co., St Louis, p. 568.

not necessarily coexist with pelvic relaxation. This point is especially true during more recent times owing to the lower parity of women. Vaginal hysterectomy is still feasible in a large number of these patients, however, even in the absence of good uterine descensus. Several leading gynecologic surgeons over the years have pointed out the feasibility of vaginal hysterectomy without good uterine descensus in selected patients. Nichols and Randall stated that "provided the uterus is moveable, the less the prolapse the easier the hysterectomy."[2] Allen and Peterson in 1954 expressed the same view.[1] These surgeons pointed to the fact that the anatomic relations and supports of such uteri are more normal and predictable.

As stressed in previous chapters, when anticipating a potentially difficult vaginal hysterectomy the final decision as to approach should be made during the examination under anesthesia. In the patient with good uterine mobility and a "roomy" pelvis, a relative lack of uterine descensus creates little difficulty. If the normal-size uterus and cervix descend at least reasonably close to the introitus, the vaginal hysterectomy should likewise be straightforward. It is when the uterine cervix cannot be readily pulled down that the situation must be carefully assessed, with the knowledge that a vaginal hysterectomy will undoubtedly be at least somewhat more difficult. If the uterus is not mobile, the bony pelvis is small, or there is a contraindication to morcellation of the uterus, an abdominal hysterectomy may be a more reasonable approach.

A laparoscopically assisted vaginal hysterectomy, as described in Chapter 3, may be considered as an alternate approach in such patients. Division of the infundibulopelvic or utero-ovarian ligaments as well as the broad ligaments may be accomplished laparoscopically before proceeding with the vaginal approach. With this technique, the surgeon must be cautious about exerting traction on the cervix as the uterine artery pedicles are approached.

The surgeon may decide to struggle transvaginally in the face of a lack of descensus when the patient is obese or otherwise medically compromised. If there is a relative lack of descensus and a relatively confining soft tissue space, the surgeon may elect to perform an episiotomy or Schuchardt incision (Fig. 6-1) to facilitate the transvaginal approach. If the relative lack of descensus appears to be secondary to an enlarged uterine fundus, the surgeon must decide whether the patient is a good candidate for transvaginal morcellation as discussed in Chapter 5. As in the patient with the enlarged uterus, when considering a transvaginal approach for a patient with a relative lack of uterine descensus, it should be apparent to the surgeon that he or she can progress to the level of ligation and transection of the uterine artery pedicles with little difficulty. Adhesions or scarring from previous pelvic disease or surgery may

Figure 6-1. Schuchardt incision. The perineal and medial levator muscles are incised.

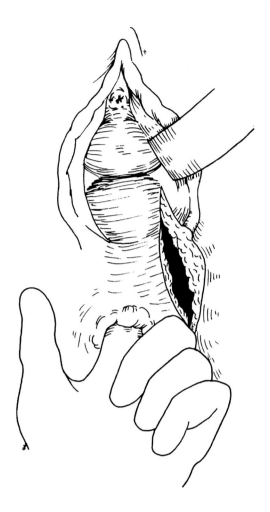

limit uterine descensus, so the patient's medical history must be considered.

As previously emphasized, it is important to have good assistance during the surgery, especially when there is minimal descensus. A few special instruments are also advantageous to the surgeon, including an extra long narrow weighted speculum, long Zeplin parametrium clamps, a long heavy needle holder, long heavy Mayo scissors, a Bovie extender, and a neurosurgery headlight (Fig. 6-2). The hysterectomy begins as outlined in Chapter 2. The posterior colpotomy will be a considerable distance from the introitus in these patients. The extra long narrow weighted speculum is advantageous here, as it can reach into the peritoneal cavity and aid immediately in exposing the uterosacral–cardinal ligament complex.

It may be advantageous to begin the operation with a posterior

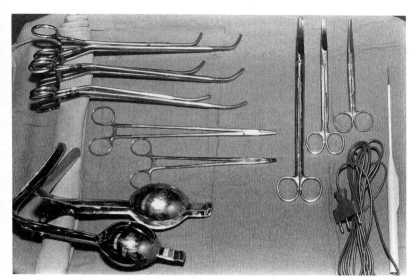

Figure 6-2. Some useful instruments for vaginal hysterectomy with lack of descensus. *Left side, top to bottom:* long and regular length Zeppelin pedicle clamps with varying angulation, long straight and regular Heaney needle holders, long narrow (regular length shown for comparison) weighted speculum. *Right side, left to right:* extra long Mayo scissors (long and regular shown for comparison) and Bovie with extender.

colpotomy and promptly clamp, cut, and ligate the uterosacral and cardinal ligaments. This maneuver often increases the amount of uterine descensus considerably, allowing access to the previously high anterior cul-de-sac. This surgically created descensus can sometimes be predicted during the examination under anesthesia and should be kept in mind when trying to decide whether a transvaginal hysterectomy is feasible. The hysterectomy may proceed easily after release of the uterosacral and cardinal ligaments; on the other hand, it may become apparent at this point or shortly thereafter that the hysterectomy can be better completed transabdominally. When the uterus still does not descend well, ligation of the subsequent pedicles becomes increasingly difficult. The surgeon may decide at this point or before to create more room in the vagina with a Schuchardt incision. The surgeon must also learn to maximize the available room by cautious manipulation of the uterus as well as dorsal, ventral, and rotational movements of the clamps while placing sutures (Figs. 6-3, 6-4).

The surgeon must proceed cautiously, taking care when applying the clamps, placing the sutures, and cutting and ligating the pedicles. There is less exposure to the pedicles than usual, consequently with less ability to compensate for errors; hence there is an overall smaller margin for error.

Figure 6-3. Pedicle clamp is cautiously moved toward the sacrum with slight rotation of the upper edge toward the operator to facilitate suture placement in a confined space.

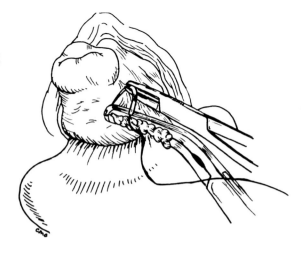

Figure 6-4. As the needle is passed under the tip, the clamp is carefully raised ventrally and the lower edge rotated slightly toward the operator to facilitate completion of suture placement.

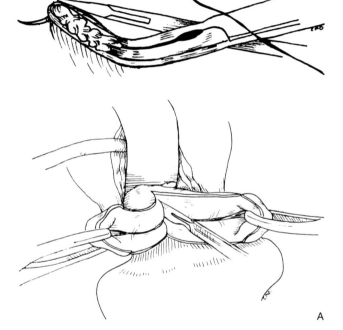

Figure 6-5. (A & B) Hemisection of the still undescended uterus is performed to facilitate exposure to the utero-ovarian pedicles.

A

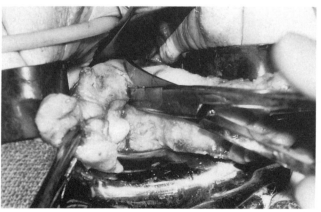

B

After ligating the uterine artery pedicles, an attempt should be made to take an additional pedicle on the broad ligaments prior to deciding that uterine manipulation or morcellation might be required. The utero-ovarian pedicles are invariably the most difficult or inaccessible pedicles to ligate in such cases. At times it is possible to place a clamp straight up across the remainder of the utero-ovarian pedicle and complete the hysterectomy in this manner. The surgeon should not struggle to accomplish this maneuver unless it is desirable to avoid morcellation. At still other times the surgeon can access these pedicles by simply amputating the cervix and flipping or rotating the fundus 180 degrees. Otherwise the best approach is to hemisect the uterus, as described in Chapter 5 (Fig. 6-5), and place one of the halves back up into the pelvis. This step creates room and exposure for the other half, affording access to its remaining utero-ovarian pedicle (Fig. 6-6). Morcellation of each half

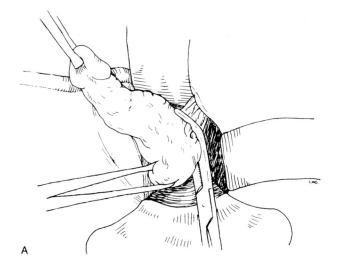

A

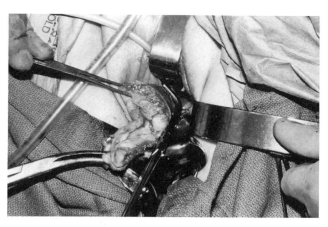

B

Figure 6-6. (A & B) Uterus has been hemisected, and half has been carefully placed back up into the pelvis. There is now good exposure to the utero-ovarian pedicle, which has been clamped.

of the hemisected uterus may be carried out if it is necessary to further improve exposure to the ligaments. The adnexae are sometimes accessible, and they should be assessed independently for removal.

References

1. Allen E, Peterson LF. Versatility of vaginal hysterectomy technique. Obstet Gynecol 3:240–247, 1954.
2. Nichols DH, Randall CL. Vaginal surgery. 3rd ed. Baltimore, Maryland. Williams and Wilkins, 1989, pp 182–238.

Suggested Reading

Barber HRK. Cystocele, urethrocele, rectocele, and enterocele. In Barber HRK, Fields DH, Kaufman SA (eds). Quick Reference to Ob-Gyn Procedures (3rd ed). Lippincott, Philadelphia, 1990, pp 356–357

Bradford WZ, Bradford WB, Woltz JHE, Brown CW. Experiences with vaginal hysterectomy. Am J Obstet Gynecol 68:540–548, 1954

Burnett LS. Relaxations, malpositions, fistulas, and incontinence. In Jones HW III, Wentz AC, Burnett LS (eds). Novak's Textbook of Gynecology (11th ed). Williams & Wilkins, Baltimore, 1988, pp 456–457

Campbell ZB. A report on 2,798 vaginal hysterectomies. Am J Obstet Gynecol 52:598–613, 1946

Davis MR. Pelvic relaxation. In Kase NG, Weingold AB, Gershenson DM (eds). Principles and Practice of Clinical Gynecology. (2nd ed). New York: Churchhill Livingstone, 1990, p 662

Dunnihoo DR. Fundamentals of Gynecology and Obstetrics. Lippincott, Philadelphia, 1990, p 57

Falk HC, Bunkin IA. A study of 500 vaginal hysterectomies. Am J Obstet Gynecol 52:623–630, 1946

Gray LA. Indications, techniques, and complications in vaginal hysterectomy. Obstet Gynecol 28:714–722, 1966

Heaney NS. A report of 565 vaginal hysterectomies performed for benign pelvic disease. Am J Obstet Gynecol 28:751–755, 1934

Isaacs JH. Vaginal hysterectomy. In Sciarra JJ, Droegemueller W (eds). Gynecology and Obstetrics (Vol 1). Lippincott, Philadelphia, 1990, pp 1–10

Käser O, Iklé FA, Hirsch HA. In Friedman EA (ed). Vaginal hysterectomy and vaginal procedures for descensus. Atlas of Gynecologic Surgery (2nd ed). Thieme-Stratton, New York, 1985

Kemp GA. The corpus uteri. In Rosenwaks Z, Benjamin F, Stone ML, (eds). Gynecology: Principles and Practice. Macmillan, New York, 1987, p 490

Kudo R, Yamauchi O, Okazaki T, et al. Vaginal hysterectomy without ligation of the ligaments of the cervix uteri. Surg Gynecol Obstet 170:299–305, 1990

Mackay EV, Beischer NA, Cox LW, Wood C. Illustrated Textbook of Gynecology. Saunders, Philadelphia, 1983, p 299

Masterson BJ. Manual of Gynecologic Surgery (2nd ed). Springer, New York, 1986, pp 108–121

Mattingly RF, Thompson JD. TeLinde's Operative Gynecology (6th ed). Lippincott, Philadelphia, 1985, pp 548–560

Netter FH. The Ciba Collection of Medical Illustrations. Vol 2. Reproductive System. Case-Hoyt Corp., Rochester, NY, 1977, p 159

Porges RF. Changing indications for vaginal hysterectomy. Am J Obstet Gynecol 136:153–158, 1980

Pratt JH, Gunnlaugsson GH. Vaginal hysterectomy by morcellation. Mayo Clin Proc 45:374–387, 1970

Sheth S, Malpani A. Vaginal hysterectomy for the management of menstruation in mentally retarded women. Int J Gynaecol Obstet 35:319–321, 1991

Stander RW. Disorders of pelvic support. In Romney SL, Gray MJ, Little AB, et al. (eds). Gynecology and Obstetrics: The Health Care of Women. McGraw-Hill, New York, 1981, p 969

Stenchever MA. Disorders of abdominal wall and pelvic support. In Droegemueller W, Herbst AL, Mishell DR Jr, Stenchever MA (eds). Comprehensive Gynecology. Mosby, St. Louis, 1987, p 530

Symmonds RE. Relaxation of pelvic supports. In Pernoll ML, Bonson RC (eds). Current Obstetric and Gynecologic Diagnosis and Treatment. Appelton & Lange, Norwalk, CT, 1987, p 760

Tovell HM, Danforth DN. Structural defects and relaxations. In Danforth DN, Scott JR, (eds). Obstetrics and Gynecology, (5th ed). Lippincott, Philadelphia, 1986, p 964

Wall LL. Disorders of pelvic support and urinary incontinence. In Clarke-Pearson DL, Dawood MY, (eds). Green's Gynecology: Essentials of Clinical Practice (4th ed). Little, Brown, Boston, 1990, pp 398–399.

Willson JR, Carrington ER, Ledger WJ, Laras RK Jr, Mattox JH. Obstetrics and Gynecology (8th ed). Mosby, St. Louis, 1987, p 568

Wynn RM. Obstetrics and Gynecology: The Clinical Core (4th ed). Lea & Febiger, Philadelphia, 1988, p 220

7

Markedly Prolapsed Uterus

The markedly prolapsed uterus lends itself well to vaginal hysterectomy. With such prolapse there is coexistent significant anatomic distortion of the urinary tract. Some technically important aspects of transvaginal removal of the markedly prolapsed uterus are described. Much of the surgical effort and therefore emphasis of this chapter is on reconstruction of genital tract anatomy and support.

Vaginal hysterectomy for mild to moderate degrees of uterine prolapse, such that with traction the cervix comes beyond the introitus, is generally straightforward. Such hysterectomies can be managed as described in Chapter 2. It is important to shorten and reattach the uterosacral–cardinal ligament complex to the vaginal cuff, close the posterior cul-de-sac, and repair associated lower genital tract defects.

When the cervix spontaneously extends beyond the introitus, a marked degree of prolapse exists, representing a significant loss of uterovaginal supports (Figs. 7-1, 7-2). In such patients the cervix frequently hypertrophies and becomes elongated, a factor that must be taken into account (Fig. 7-3). In some patients, especially when the cervix is elongated, the uterosacral ligaments are still strong enough to provide good vault support. The more severe cases of uterovaginal prolapse tend to occur in multiparous postmenopausal women. In the most severe cases, where the vagina

Figure 7-1. Uterovaginal prolapse with a prominent anterior segment defect (Baden and Walker classification[1]).

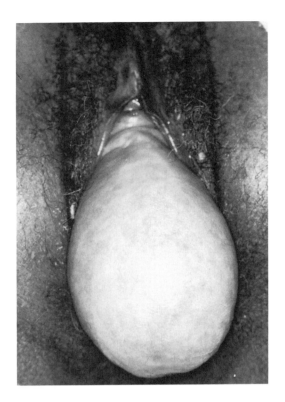

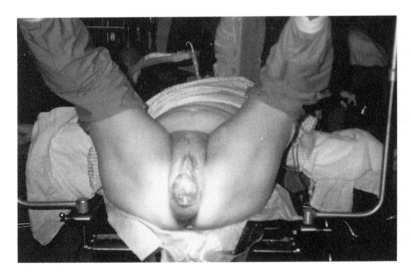

Figure 7-2. Uterovaginal prolapse with a prominent posterior segment defect.[1]

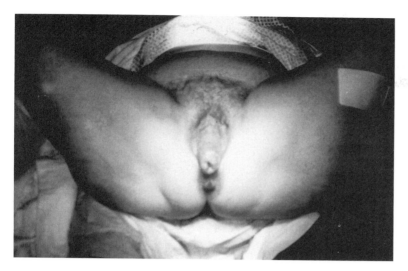

Figure 7-3. Pseudoprolapse. The cervix is markedly elongated and in this case protrudes through the vulva. The uterine fundus is higher in the pelvis, in a relatively normal position. Associated defects are variable, and the mechanism(s) by which this pseudoprolapse occurs is not entirely understood.

has completely prolapsed with the uterus, surgical correction can be technically difficult.

With longstanding severe prolapse the cervical-vaginal mucosa may be edematous, chronically inflamed, at times ulcerated, markedly thickened, and partially keratinized. These ulcerations can predispose the patient to postoperative infection. In postmenopausal women preoperative estrogen replacement therapy thickens the vaginal mucosa and improves dissection and healing. When mucosal ulcerations are present, the patient may benefit from a short course of topical antibiotics, estrogen replacement therapy, and sitz baths or warm saline soaks prior to surgery. If an isolated ulceration appears at all suspicious for malignancy it should be biopsied. Rarely, the patient presents acutely with an inability to reduce a prolapsed uterus. This situation is probably due to tissue edema and may be best managed initially with bed rest and warm saline soaks. If improvement does not occur promptly after such treatment, the patient should be taken to surgery without delay.

With uterine prolapse the vagina becomes somewhat shortened. The bladder, ureters, and at times even the urethra and rectum also become prolapsed as even the lower vaginal supports are lost (Fig. 7-4). The cervix tends to further elongate and narrow. The posterior cul-de-sac becomes a deep pocket extending out of the pelvis (Fig. 7-5). These anatomic alterations obscure the surgical planes and place them in aberrant locations, with the bladder and ureters in positions that challenge the operator to avoid them (Fig. 7-6). The difficult aspect of removing a severely prolapsed uterus lies in the circumvention of the anatomic changes so as to extirpate the uterus efficiently without incurring an injury. The most difficult

Figure 7-4. Uterovaginal prolapse. Note the prolapse of the anterior vaginal wall and loss of urethral support.

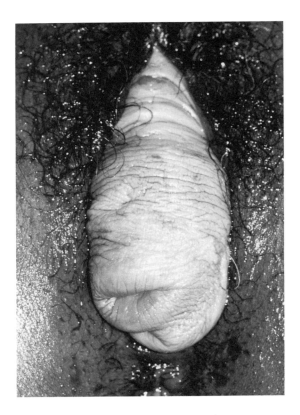

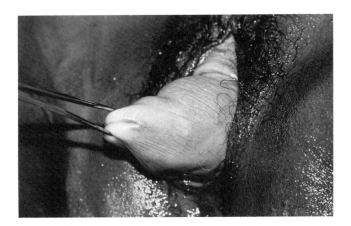

Figure 7-5. Uterovaginal prolapse with an evidently deep posterior cul-de-sac (culdocele[1]).

aspect of the surgery, however, begins after removal of the uterus. Reconstruction of support for the remaining prolapsed organs requires extensive surgical effort and should be the main focus of the operation. This chapter describes the technical aspects of safe removal of the severely prolapsed uterus and outlines some methods for dealing with the remaining prolapsed vagina.

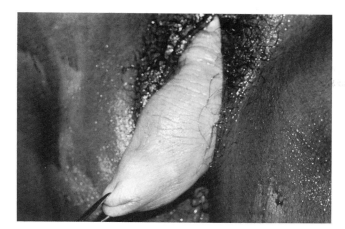

Figure 7-6. Portion of the bladder has prolapsed with the uterus and vagina. The operator must be knowledgeable about and aware of this anatomic relation so as to avoid injury to the urinary tract.

Preoperative Evaluation

For the patient with longstanding severe uterovaginal prolapse, an intravenous pyelogram should be considered preoperatively to evaluate the condition of the upper urinary tracts. It is not unusual for such patients to have some element of hydroureteronephrosis. Utilization of urodynamic evaluation in these patients is complicated by the marked difference in the pre- and postoperative positions of the bladder and urethra. Several studies have reported good results after temporarily replacing the cervix or the top of the vagina back into its normal position during the urodynamic evaluation. Even when this is done however, it should be kept in mind that most of these patients have significant defects of the anterior vaginal wall supports that require correction. The preoperative assessment should also include a careful pelvic examination to determine the degree of coexistent loss of upper and lower vaginal supports.

Vaginal Hysterectomy

The vaginal hysterectomy is carried out for the most part, in a straightforward manner, as described in Chapter 2. If there is much edema and thickening of the vaginal mucosa, the cervix may be difficult to palpate, particularly when it is elongated and thin. The mucosa should be circumscribed close to the cervical os in order to avoid injury to the prolapsed bladder and to preserve vaginal length. The soft tissue containing the bladder and ureters is mobilized off the cervix and proximal parametria. The anterior and posterior peritoneal reflections may be relatively high owing to cervical elongation. Early mobilization of the anterior and lateral soft tissues and elevation of the bladder off the cervix with a retractor helps to avoid bladder and ureteral injury. If difficulty is encountered, inci-

Figure 7-7. (A & B) Anterior vaginal mucosa is incised from the cervix to the urethra and is then dissected off the cervix and bladder. The demarcation between the uterus and bladder is now more evident.

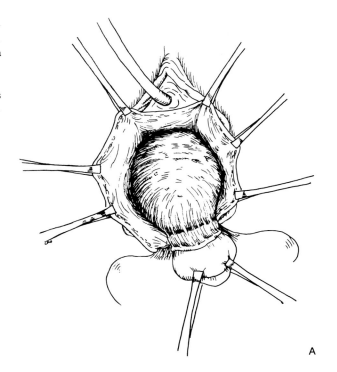

A

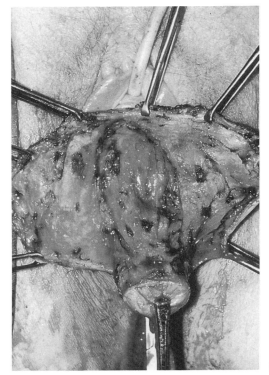

B

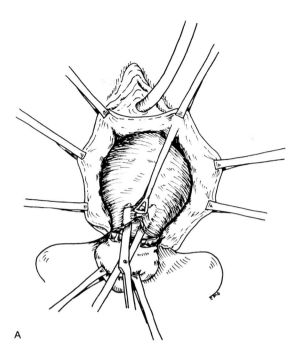

A

Figure 7-8. (A & B) Bladder is dissected from the cervix to the peritoneal reflection. This dissection should be cautiously extended laterally from the midline just far enough to ensure safe ligation of the paracervical tissues away from the bladder and ureters.

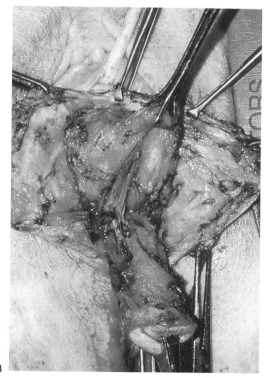

B

sion of the anterior vaginal wall and mobilization of the vaginal mucosal flaps laterally give the operator more room in which to work and a better idea of the location of the bladder (Figs. 7-7, 7-8). The same may be done posteriorly as the operator attempts to locate the posterior cul-de-sac. If the posterior cul-de-sac can be entered early, it may further help to orient the surgeon, making it easier to locate the correct plane of dissection and avoid urinary tract injury.

When the cervix is markedly elongated, the cardinal ligaments are, at least at their inferior portion, elongated and thinned out (Fig. 7-9). Several pedicles may be clamped before the uterine artery pedicles are reached. Only the uppermost of these pedicles should be used for reattachment to the vaginal cuff. If the soft tissue can be mobilized laterally and the surgeon is confident of the anatomic landmarks, ligation of the cardinal ligaments can begin a little higher. The inferior portion of markedly elongated and thinned cardinal ligaments and bladder pillars may be divided at the cervix with cautery. In the presence of hydroureters, particular care must be taken to mobilize the anterior and lateral soft tissues and to keep all clamps close to the cervix. Once the prolapsed bladder has been mobilized off the cervix, as shown in Figures 7-8 and 7-9, the surgeon can palpate the ureter in the bladder pillar (vesicouterine ligament) prior to clamping the inferior pedicles (Fig. 7-10).

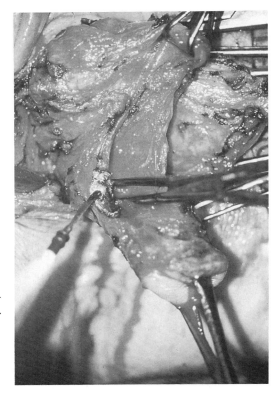

Figure 7-9. Bladder has been dissected free of the vagina and the elongated cervix. Markedly elongated, thinned ligamentous tissue appears along the lateral edge of this cervix. Some of this tissue is being divided with cautery.

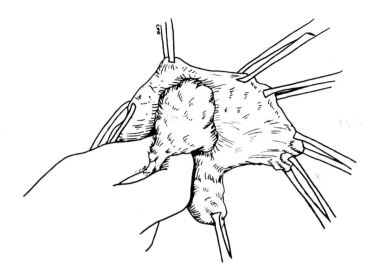

Figure 7-10. With one finger under the bladder base and one finger between the bladder and the anterior vaginal flap, the ureter is often palpable in the elongated vesicouterine ligament (bladder pillar). Such palpation is reassuring during ligation of the paracervical tissues.

Once the anterior and posterior cul-de-sacs have been entered and the uterine artery pedicles ligated, the hysterectomy is completed easily. High purse-string closure of the peritoneal defect with permanent suture should be performed to prevent a future enterocele. A second reinforcing purse-string suture should also be placed. The work of reconstructing the vaginal supports then begins.

Planning Reconstruction

The first step in the reconstruction of vaginal supports is assessment of the anterior vaginal wall and vaginal cuff supports. The uterosacral–cardinal ligament complex has been surgically shortened somewhat and was reattached to the vaginal cuff as these pedicles were ligated. In the presence of marked uterovaginal prolapse, however, it is unlikely that this will provide adequate vaginal vault support.

If reasonably identifiable and strong uterosacral ligaments are present (Fig. 7-11), they can be used effectively to support the vaginal cuff. A high stitch can be placed using long Babcock or Allis clamps to identify the insertion of these ligaments higher in the pelvis toward the sacrum. When placed in the manner of a modified McCall's culdoplasty this stitch simultaneously obliterates the posterior cul-de-sac and brings the vagina into its proper axis, preventing a future enterocele and vault prolapse (see Fig. 2-14). Caution is warranted when placing this stitch, as the uterosacral ligaments may be difficult to identify at this point and the ureters generally traverse within a short distance lateral to them. Prior to tying this culdoplasty stitch the high purse-string closure of the peritoneal defect

Figure 7-11. (A & B)
Outward and upward traction
on these cervices demon-
strates elongated but visible
and palpably strong uterosacral ligaments.

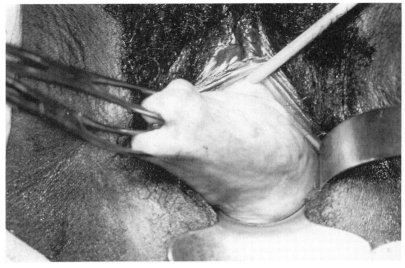

A

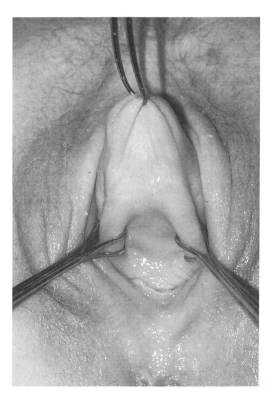

B

is performed, and anterior and posterior colporrhaphy is carried out as appropriate. If there are no surgically usable uterosacral ligaments and the vaginal cuff is in need of further support, it can be attached to the sacrospinous ligament–coccygeus muscle complex.

Sacrospinous Colpopexy

Sacrospinous Colpopexy has been advocated by Nichols and Randall[5] and supported in a study done by Cruikshank and colleagues.[2,3] A high purse-string closure of the peritoneal defect is accomplished, and the cuff is initially left open. A full-length anterior colporrhaphy is then performed. The perineum and full length of the posterior vaginal wall are incised in preparation for the perineorrhaphy and posterior colporrhaphy. The vaginal flaps are dissected laterally. For the right-handed operator the right vaginal flap is dissected all the way to the right posterior vaginal sulcus and off the perineal body. With further blunt dissection pararectally, the puborectalis muscle is exposed above the perineal body occupying its normal position along the lateral aspect of the lower vagina. With further blunt dissection just lateral to the rectum above the puborectalis muscle, the right rectal pillars are encountered. This tissue, extending laterally from the rectum to the pelvic side wall is relatively avascular connective tissue that can be perforated with little affort. Using the index and middle fingers of the right hand the

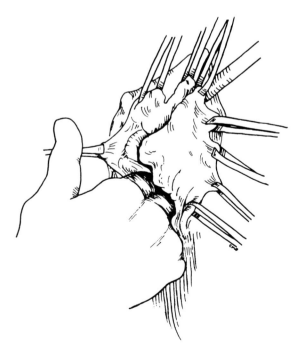

Figure 7-12. Blunt digital dissection is performed toward the ischial spine to develop the pararectal space and expose the coccygeus muscle.

surgeon generally can perform blunt dissection cautiously through this tissue toward the ischial spine (Fig. 7-12).

Once broken through, the fingers are spread and the tissue with the rectum is bluntly mobilized medially toward the sacrum in order to expose the sacrospinal ligament–coccygeus muscle complex. Occasionally the tissue is dense, and a blunt instrument can be used to gain access to this space. Once opened, retractors are placed so as to provide direct visualization of the ligament–muscle complex. Two Breisky-Navratil retractors are useful for superior and medial retraction (Fig. 7-13). Care must be taken not to retract across the vascular presacral area. The notched retractor, which is sold in conjunction with the Miya hook, is used posterolaterally just inferior to

Figure 7-13. Some useful instruments for sacrospinous colpopexy. *Top, left to right:* bovie, Miya hook, tonsil clamp, notched Miya hook retractor. *Middle:* No. 1 or 2 delayed absorbable or permanent suture and free Mayo needle. *Bottom:* Two Breisky-Navratil retractors.

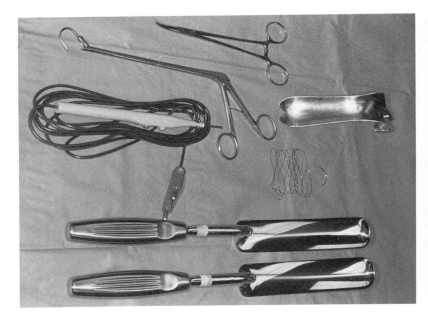

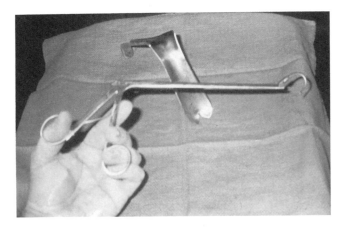

Figure 7-14. Miya hook in "opened" position and retractor. The tip of the hook (with suture) is placed against the superior edge of the muscle to include approximately one-third of its thickness (in a ventral to dorsal direction) and then squeezed closed.

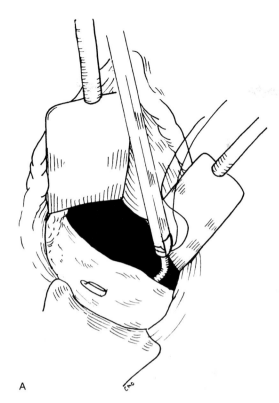

Figure 7-15. (A & B) Hook is pulled through the muscle at this level until its tip is seen exiting the inferior edge. The suture is retrieved from the tip with a tonsil or nerve hook, and the Miya hook is then backed out (still squeezed close). Once out of the muscle the handle is released, the instrument withdrawn, and the end of the suture freed.

A

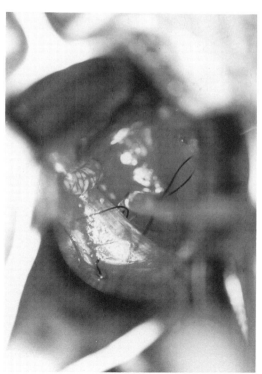

B

the ligament (Fig. 7-14). This retractor is placed in the space and withdrawn slowly while exerting firm pressure until the ligament–muscle complex rolls up in front of the retractor.

Using the Miya hook, a No. 1 polypropylene or polydioxanone suture is placed through approximately the anterior one-third of the ligament–muscle complex (Fig. 7-15). The suture should be placed 2 to 3 cm medial to the ischial spine to avoid injury to the sciatic nerve and pudendal vessels. Placement of the Miya hook retractor as described generally ensure this safety. The loop of suture is grasped from the Miya hook with a tonsil clamp or nerve hook and pulled through, and the Miya hook is withdrawn. The end of the loop is cut and the ends of each suture matched to provide two sutures through the ligament with one throw (Fig. 7-16). While the Miya hook is in place, moderate traction is applied to ensure a good purchase. These sutures are tagged and held without tying, and hemostasis is ensured.

The posterior vaginal mucosa is then trimmed. A minimal amount of mucosa is excised from the upper part of the posterior vagina, especially on the right side to ensure that the vaginal cuff will reach the sacrospinous ligament and to maintain a capacious vaginal vault. When the sutures are tied, they have a further narrowing effect on the vagina; and if too much upper vaginal mucosa is excised, the patient is left with a rather narrow upper tube directed toward the right side. On the other hand, as pointed out by Nichols and Randall,[5] leaving too much upper vagina can predispose to a recurrence of the prolapse.

After trimming the posterior vaginal mucosa, a free Mayo needle is used to place an end of each of the polypropylene sutures through the submucosa of the right vaginal flap near the posterior

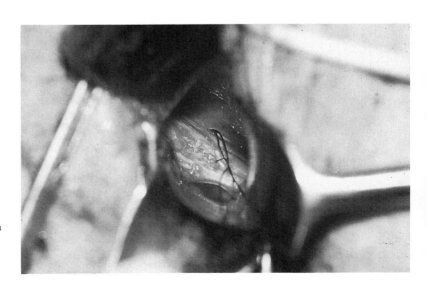

Figure 7-16. Miya hook has been withdrawn. Traction is placed on the sutures (two strands together) in the ligament–muscle complex.

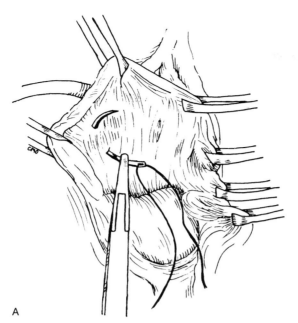

Figure 7-17. (A & B) One end of each of the two stitches is placed through a selected site in the vaginal mucosa or submucosa with a free Mayo needle.

A

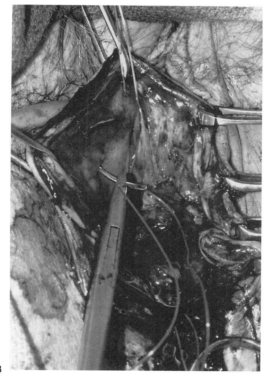

B

apex (Fig. 7-17). Using an Allis clamp, the surgeon should ensure that this part of the vagina can readily reach the ligament. A long bite extending close to but not through (with permanent suture) the mucosa should be placed to ensure a good supporting suture. If the vagina is thin, an additional delayed absorbable suture can be placed through the ligament and full thickness of the vagina. These sutures are again held without tying. It is helpful to tie a single throw of the portion of suture entering and exiting the vaginal submucosa (Fig. 7-18). It creates a "pulley" stitch, which allows the surgeon to test the correctness of the placement and makes final tying of the sutures easier and more precise. When the other end of the pulley stitch is gently tractioned, the vaginal cuff should readily ascend to the coccygeus muscle without tension and create the desired anatomic effect.

If a rectocele repair is to be performed, it should be done at this time. If puborectalis plication stitches are placed, however, they should not be tied until the entire procedure is almost completed. It is our habit to plicate at least the inferior portion of the puborectalis muscles to the midline with polydioxanone sutures. The superior portion of the perineal body may be included in this stitch as described by Nichols.[4] This plication narrows the widened genital hiatus and reinforces the levator plate. The upper vagina, which has been placed back into the hollow of the sacrum by the sacrospinous colpopexy, is resting on and supported by this reinforced shelf. With adequate mobilization of the rectum, the stitches can be placed more dorsally (Fig. 7-19), which avoids a vaginal shelf

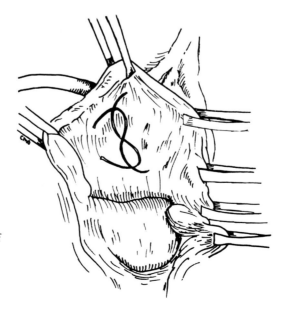

Figure 7-18. A single throw is placed on the part of the suture entering and exiting the vaginal submucosa in order to create the "pulley" stitch.

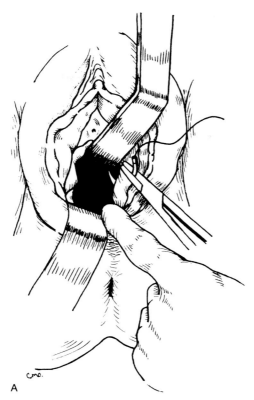

Figure 7-19. (A & B)
Rectum has been mobilized
off the posterior vaginal wall
and puborectalis muscles.
The left posterior vaginal wall
is being retracted ventrally
with a Heaney retractor, and
the rectum is being retracted
medially with a Deaver retractor, exposing the medial
aspect of the left puborectalis
muscle. The stitch being
placed into the left muscle
will be brought across to the
right muscle for plication to
the midline while avoiding a
vaginal ridge or rectal narrowing. Several such sutures
may be placed at the discre-
tion of the surgeon.

A

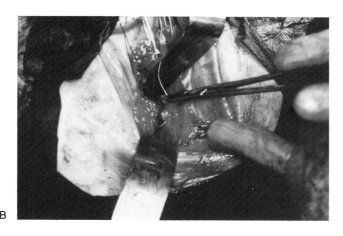

B

with its attendant potential for dyspareunia. The surgeon must
check that the rectum has not been unduly narrowed.

The vaginal cuff and posterior vaginal wall closures are begun
using a running interlocking stitch of delayed absorbable suture
that is carried to approximately the mid-vagina. The sacrospinous
sutures are then tied, ensuring direct approximation of the upper
vagina to the ligament–muscle complex (the pulley mechanism

helps with this step). Closure of the vaginal mucosa is completed, and a perineorrhaphy is carried out. The surgeon must be certain that the vaginal depth is adequate for sexual relations. A vaginal pack is placed and then removed in approximately 24 hours.

Anterior Vaginal Wall Prolapse

Patients with marked uterine prolapse often have coexistent marked prolapse of the anterior vaginal wall. The latter is generally a midline defect due to stretching of the anterior vaginal wall or a prolapse of the upper anterior vaginal wall that has resulted from loss of upper vaginal support. Such defects are repaired, as previously described above, by anterior colporrhaphy and resupporting the vaginal vault. Some patients, however, have a coexistent paravaginal defect as a result of loss of the fibrous attachments of the anterolateral portions of the mid-vagina to the arcus tendineus. This defect is identified when there is a relative absence of the anterior vaginal sulci in their normal position evidencing loss of the lateral supports of the mid-anterior vaginal wall. When examining the patient for this defect, it is helpful to replace the uterus and upper vagina into the anticipated final reconstructed position (Fig. 7-20). When there is a coexistent paravaginal defect, repair with an anterior colporrhaphy

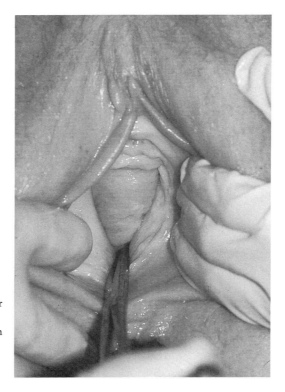

Figure 7-20. Prolapsed uterus has been placed back into the pelvis with the upper vagina at the anticipated reconstructed site. Examination of the anterior vaginal wall now demonstrates a large midline defect.

and resupport of the vaginal vault may leave the patient prone to persistent or recurrent anterior vaginal wall prolapse.

Paravaginal Defect

In the patient undergoing surgical correction for marked uterovaginal prolapse, a paravaginal defect should be carefully sought and, if present, repaired at the time of hysterectomy. Currently, there are two well described techniques for this repair. One technique consists of reattaching the lateral portions of the mid-anterior vaginal wall to the arcus tendineus by direct suturing, which is generally done via access to the space of Retzius through an abdominal incision. The technique may also be performed transvaginally, as originally described by White[7] in 1909 and later by Nichols and Randall[5] and Baden and Walker.[1] When operating vaginally to correct prolapse, we have preferred to correct a paravaginal defect by a slight modification of the four-corner needle suspension described by Raz.[6] This technique combines a needle suspension of the bladder neck (two of the corners) with a needle suspension of the mid and upper anterior vaginal wall (the other two corners).

Four-Corner Needle Suspension

The four-corner needle suspension is begun after completing the hysterectomy. It is helpful to have tagged the cardinal ligament pedicles. If a McCall's culdoplasty stitch is placed, it should not be tied until the anterior vaginal repair has been completed. If a sacrospinous colpopexy is also planned, this stitch should be placed and held without tying prior to tying the polypropylene bladder suspension sutures. If the anterior vaginal wall has not yet been incised, it is done in the midline from the anterior vaginal cuff to approximately 1 cm from the urethral meatus.

The vaginal mucosal flaps are separated from the bladder and bladder neck (Fig. 7-7). Superiorly, this separation is carried to the previously tagged cardinal ligament pedicles. It is important to separate the upper urethra and bladder neck beyond their attachments to the vaginal mucosa prior to attempting dissection into the space of Retzius. While applying countertraction with Allis clamps on the vaginal mucosa, at the level of the proximal urethra the index finger is directed lateral to the bladder neck against the underside of the pubic symphysis. Using short, sweeping movements, the index finger continues to push the soft tissues medially as they are encountered, guided by a path of least resistance. The general direction is toward the patient's ipsilateral shoulder. A distinct "give" finally releases the finger into the space of Retzius. Further mobilization of the tissues around this opening may lead to troublesome bleeding and should be avoided. Finger dissection not directed laterally enough may result in troublesome venous plexus bleeding or injury to the bladder neck.

After dissection into the space of Retzius on both sides, a triple helical stitch is placed on each side of the bladder with No. 0 poly-propylene suture. Judging which area of the vagina will reside just lateral to the proximal urethra and bladder neck after trimming and closure, the stitches are placed through the submucosa (as thick as possible) starting at either the level of the proximal urethra or about 1 to 2 cm above the bladder neck. The stitch is passed back and forth from the vaginal submucosal fascia to the lateral periurethral and perivesical "fascia" at three consecutive sites (proximal urethra, bladder neck, and 1 to 2 cm above the bladder neck) (Fig. 7-21). If strong tissue immediately lateral to the urethra can be identified (i.e., pubourethral ligament) that elevates the proximal urethra when tractioned, it may be preferable to use this tissue rather than the side of the urethra. After traction is applied to these polypropy-lene sutures, the urethra may be distorted along its lateral wall, which theoretically could lead to a scarred, low-pressure urethra.

After the two bladder neck sutures have been placed and tagged, an additional triple helical polypropylene stitch is placed into the mid to upper lateral anterior vaginal submucosa on each side, with the highest bite being taken through the previously tagged cardinal ligament pedicle (Fig. 7-22). These sutures are held long with dif-ferent instruments from the bladder neck sutures.

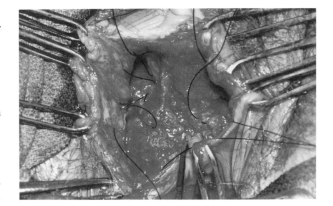

Figure 7-21. Vagina has been dissected off the bladder neck and is held with Allis clamps. On the right side of the bladder neck, the begin-ning of the opening into the space of Retzius can be seen. A triple helical stitch has been placed on both sides, extend-ing from just above to just below the bladder neck. The stitch shown here includes vaginal submucosa and corre-sponding periurethral/perive-sical tissue. Alternatively, the surgeon may elect to include the vaginal submucosa only (for needle colposuspension) and separately plicate the periurethral/perivesical tissues to the midline.

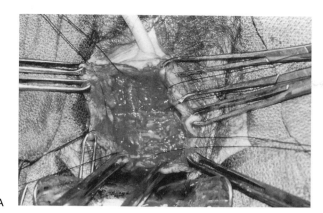

Figure 7-22. (A & B) In addition to the two stitches placed lateral to the bladder neck, two more triple helical sutures have been placed, designed to suspend the upper anterior vaginal wall. These sutures are placed according to the individual defect and anatomy but, in general, extend from the mid-anterior vagina to the cardinal ligament pedicle.

A

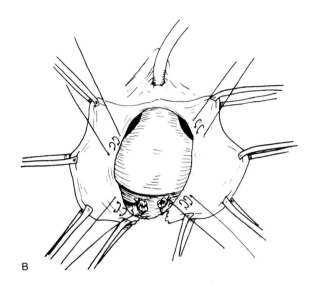

B

A small transverse incision (2 to 3 cm depending on the size of the patient) is then made just at the superior border of the pubic symphysis in the midline, carried down to the rectus fascia. With the bladder neck sutures held loosely, an index finger is placed above the most superior helical throw and back into the space of Retzius. Using this finger to displace the bladder neck safely away, a Stamey needle is brought through the abdominal wound toward the side of the finger (Fig. 7-23A). The Stamey needle should puncture the fascia close to the pubic symphysis. After the needle is through the fascia it is readily felt with the finger and guided into the vaginal opening (Fig. 7-23B). The two ends of the polypropylene suture on the same side of the bladder neck are threaded through the eye of the Stamey needle and pulled back through the abdominal wound. The ends are held with a hemostat. The procedure is then repeated on the opposite side. Just lateral to these sites

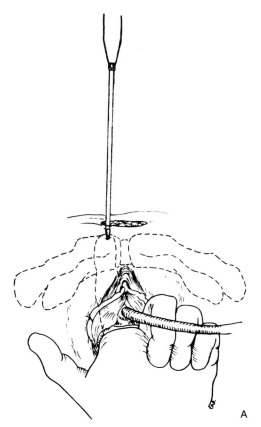

A

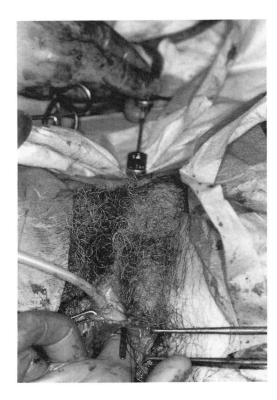

B

Figure 7-23. (A & B) The surgeon's index finger has been placed retropubically into the space of Retzius. The finger simultaneously is applied against the rectus fascia while dispacing the bladder neck safely away. Once through the fascia, the Stamey needle is palpated and guided into the vagina.

on the rectus fascia, the Stamey needle is reintroduced back into the vaginal incision. On the respective side, the upper vaginal polypropylene suture (both ends) is threaded and pulled back into the abdominal incision. This stitch is held with a different clamp (straight hemostat). The suture on the opposite side is likewise pulled through and tagged.

A midline cystocele plication is then performed. If significant stress urinary incontinence exists, consideration may be given to additionally plicating the bladder neck and urethra to the midline with the pubourethral ligaments or other available tissues. If this type of bladder neck plication is planned, the surgeon may consider placing the helical polypropylene bladder neck suspension sutures through the vaginal submucosa only (colposuspension) (Fig. 7-22B).

At this time, 5 ml of indigo carmine is administered intravenously. The Foley catheter is separated from the drainage tube, and the bladder is completely emptied. The bladder is then filled with approximately 200 ml of saline and the catheter removed. A cystoscope with a 70-degree lens is introduced. The urethra and bladder (particularly the bladder neck area) are inspected to be certain that the polypropylene sutures do not traverse intraluminally. The ureteral orifices are visualized to be sure dye is spurting from each, without and with tension on the bladder neck sutures. Switching to a 0-degree cystoscope, the bladder neck is observed while applying tension to both bladder neck sutures (to elevate the bladder neck). Traction on properly placed bladder neck sutures should readily bring about closure of the bladder neck lumen. Excess vaginal mucosa is then trimmed, and the vagina is closed with a running lock 2-0 delayed absorbable suture (the vaginal cuff may be left open with the edges sutured).

The polypropylene suspension sutures are now tied (Fig. 7-24). If the four-corner procedure has been utilized, the superior sutures are

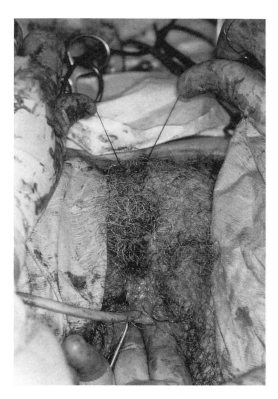

Figure 7-24. Traction on the sutures readily elevates the bladder neck (unless a midline plication has been done).

tied first. These sutures are intended to pull the sagging anterior vaginal wall away from the introitus, but care should be taken not to overcorrect beyond the normal position of the anterior vaginal wall and bladder. If desired, the sutures on each side may be tied separately by taking a bite of fascia with a free needle. The two strands from one side should still be tied across the midline to the strands from the other side for extra security.

The bladder neck suspension sutures are then tied. The optimal method of determining how tight to tie these sutures is not well established. We use a combination of a sterile Q-tip and urethro-scopy. The Q-tip is placed into the bladder and pulled back to the bladder neck. The suspension sutures are tractioned until the Q-tip becomes horizontal relative to the supine patient. At this level of tension we assess the effect on bladder neck closure with the cysto-scope. The sutures should not be tied with great tension, as it may lead to urinary retention postoperatively and later to failure of the suspension.

The suprapubic wound is then thoroughly irrigated with 1 liter of bacitracin solution (50,000 units) and closed with interrupted verti-cal mattress sutures or skin staples. Our policy is to remove the Foley catheter on postoperative day 3 and check a postvoid resid-ual urine volume after the second void.

Vaginectomy

When the elderly patient with severe uterovaginal prolapse under-goes vaginal hysterectomy and there is clearly no desire to retain the capacity for intercourse, another option for management of the remaining prolapsed vagina is vaginectomy. This procedure may not save any operative time or blood loss, may not be optimal in terms of future local organ function, and overall is probably little more effective than retaining the vagina with the above procedures. Surgi-cal judgment indicates which procedure is best for the patient.

After vaginal hysterectomy closure of the peritoneal defect is ac-complished with a high purse-string suture. It is prudent to perform extensive closure of the cul-de-sac, as vaginectomy does not neces-sarily prevent a future enterocele. The lower one-third of the vagina is preserved for purposes of the urethral and low rectal support. A circumferential incision is made at this level, and the remainder of the vagina is excised in quadrants. Any cystocele or rectocele is repaired and the urethrovesicle angle plicated. The puborectalis muscles are also extensively plicated to the midline anterior to the rectum, and the upper portion of the remaining posterior vaginal stump is attached to these muscles. Serial purse-string sutures are placed to the upper bladder and upper rectum in a superior to inferior direction as their prolapse is reduced and they are replaced back into a relatively normal position. The vaginal stump is then closed.

References

1. Baden WF, Walker T. The anatomy of uterovaginal support. In Baden WF, Walker T (eds). Surgical Repair of Vaginal Defects. Lippincott, Philadelphia, 1991, pp 25–50
2. Cruikshank SH. Sacrospinous fixation—should this be performed at the time of vaginal hysterectomy? Am J Obstet Gynecol 164:1072–1076, 1991
3. Cruikshank SH, Cox DW. Sacrospinous ligament fixation at the time of transvaginal hysterectomy. Am J Obstet Gynecol 162:1611–1619, 1990
4. Nichols DH. Sacrospinous fixation for massive eversion of the vagina. Am J Obstet Gynecol 142:901–904, 1982
5. Nichols DH, Randall CL. Vaginal Surgery. (3rd ed). Williams & Wilkins, Baltimore, 1989, pp 182–238
6. Raz S. Atlas of Transvaginal Surgery. Saunders, Philadelphia, 1992, pp 66–77
7. White GR. Cystocele. JAMA 53:1707, 1909

Suggested Reading

Allen E, Peterson LF. Versatility of vaginal hysterectomy technique. Obstet Gynecol 3:240–247, 1954

Bergman A, Koonings PP, Ballard CA. Predicting postoperative urinary incontinence development in women undergoing operation for genitourinary prolapse. Am J Obstet Gynecol 158:1171–1175, 1988

Bump RC, Fantl JA, Hurt WG. The mechanism of urinary incontinence in women with severe uterovaginal prolapse: results of barrier studies. Obstet Gynecol 72:291–295, 1988

Campbell ZB. A report on 2,798 vaginal hysterectomies. Am J Obstet Gynecol 52:598–613, 1946

Copenhaver EH. Vaginal hysterectomy: an analysis of indication and complications among 1,000 operations. Am J Obstet Gynecol 84:123–128, 1962

Cruikshank SH. Preventing posthysterectomy vaginal vault prolapse and enterocele during vaginal hysterectomy. Am J Obstet Gynecol 156:1433–1440, 1987

Cruikshank SH, Kovac SR. Anatomic changes of ureter during vaginal hysterectomy. Contemp Obstet Gynecol February:38–53, 1993

Given FT Jr. "Posterior culdoplasty": revisited. Am J Obstet Gynecol 153:135–139, 1985

Gray LA. Indications, techniques, and complications in vaginal hysterectomy. Obstet Gynecol 28:714–722, 1966

Heaney NS. A report of 565 vaginal hysterectomies performed for benign pelvic disease. Am J Obstet Gynecol 28:751–755, 1934

Käser O, Iklé FA, Hirsch HA. In Friedman EA (ed). Vaginal hysterectomy and vaginal procedures for descensus. Atlas of Gynecologic Surgery (2nd ed). Thieme-Stratton, New York, 1985

Langmade CF, Oliver JA Jr. Partial colpocleisis. Am J Obstet Gynecol 154:1200–1205, 1986

Mattingly RF, Thompson JD. TeLinde's Operative Gynecology (6th ed). Lippincott, Philadelphia, 1985, pp 548–560

McCall ML. Posterior culdoplasty: surgical correction of enterocele during vaginal hysterectomy; a preliminary report. Am J Obstet Gynecol 10:595–602, 1957

Miyazaki FS. Miya hook ligature carrier for sacrospinous ligament suspension. Obstet Gynecol 70:286–288, 1987

Nichols DH. Vaginal prolapse affecting bladder function. Urol Clin North Am 12:329–338, 1985

Rosenzweig BA, Blumenfeld D, Bhatia NN. Incidence of urinary incontinence in asymptomatic women with severe genitourinary prolapse: a rationale for preoperative urodynamic evaluation [abstract]. In Proceedings of the Annual ACOG Meeting, 1991

Reiffenstuhl G, Platzer W, Friedman EA (eds). Atlas of Vaginal Surgery: Surgical Anatomy and Technique (Vol 1). Saunders, Philadelphia, 1975, pp 286–301

TeLinde RW. Prolapse of the uterus and allied conditions. Am J Obstet Gyencol 94:444–463, 1966

Word BH Jr, Baden WF, Montgomery HA, Walker T. Vaginal approach to anterior paravaginal repair: alternative techniques. In Baden WF, Walker T (eds). Surgical Repair of Vaginal Defects. Philadelphia, Lippincott, 1992, pp 195–207

8

Prior Pelvic Surgery

A history of pelvic surgery has been a source of concern when considering a patient for vaginal hysterectomy. Postsurgical scarring and adhesions may produce relative fixation of the uterus or adherence of the urinary or intestinal tract with resultant predisposition to injury. The nature and relative risk of problems associated with some of the commonly encountered prior pelvic operations are discussed. Some methods of transvaginally managing a variety of potentially complicated postsurgical changes are described. When good uterine mobility and other anatomic factors favorable for vaginal hysterectomy are present, significant difficulties related to the prior pelvic surgery are unlikely. A cautious approach is of course warranted.

Prior pelvic surgery has been considered by some gynecologists to be a relative or even an absolute contraindication to vaginal hysterectomy, although several reasonably large reports have indicated the feasibility and safety of vaginal hysterectomy in most of these patients. In 1973 Coulam and Pratt published a report of 621 patients with histories of previous pelvic surgery who underwent vaginal hysterectomy.[2] In no case was there failure to complete the vaginal hysterectomy. In addition, the 621 patients were compared to 942 vaginal hysterectomy patients who had not undergone previous pelvic surgery, and there was no difference in the complication rates.

Several other studies have confirmed these results. Indeed, there are no significant data in the literature that refute the safety and feasibility of vaginal hysterectomy in patients who have previously undergone pelvic surgery. Most of the studies pertaining to this issue, as well as some recent surgical textbooks, state that the decision on the route of hysterectomy should be based on uterine mobility, pelvic architecture, and other such factors as discussed in Chapter 2 and be independent of the history of prior pelvic surgery.

It is difficult to speak in general terms about the effect of prior pelvic surgery on the feasibility of vaginal hysterectomy. The gynecologic surgeon is aware that certain types of previous pelvic surgery are likely to alter the pelvic anatomy significantly. Thus the surgeon must consider certain questions when approaching such a patient.

Do the anatomic changes that may have been caused by the prior surgery predispose the patient to an increased risk of urinary or intestinal tract injury during hysterectomy?

Does the route of the hysterectomy alter this risk?

Are there anatomic alterations that may make the vaginal or the abdominal route preferable?

The gynecologic surgeon must be concerned not only with the particular prior surgery reported by the patient but also with any complications that may have occurred and the findings at the time of surgery, including the nature and extent of any disease process that might have been encountered.

Some previous reports have included distant abdominal surgery, such as cholecystectomy and appendectomy, in their analysis of vaginal hysterectomy after previous pelvic surgery. This type of surgery generally should have little or no bearing on later pelvic surgery. For example, in the report by Coulam and Pratt, 514 of the 866 prior surgeries were appendectomies.[2] Campbell reported vaginal hysterectomy after appendectomy in 339 patients.[1] Neither of these studies reported any significant problems with the vaginal hysterectomy. If a patient is known to have had complicated appendicitis with a ruptured appendix or a periappendiceal abscess, especially if the abscess or bowel adhesions involved the uterus, the gynecologic surgeon would need to be more cautious about choosing the vaginal route for hysterectomy.

The literature reveals that partial or complete adnexectomy, uterine suspension, and cesarean section are the most common prior gynecologic operations performed in patients who subsequently underwent vaginal hysterectomy. Some of the other pelvic operations included laparotomy only, abscess drainage, colporrhaphy, and myomectomy.

Prior Adnexal Surgery

Based on published reports, partial or complete removal of the adnexa does not pose any significant obstacle to vaginal hysterectomy. However, as noted previously, the surgeon must consider the operative findings and the nature and extent of any disease process noted at the previous surgery. If the previous adnexal surgery was performed for severe endometriosis or pelvic inflammatory disease, a subsequent vaginal hysterectomy may be difficult or hazardous. The latter is especially true if there has been extensive involvement or obliteration of the anterior or posterior cul-de-sac or if extensive intestinal adhesions have formed to the uterus.

Uterine Suspension

A prior uterine suspension is one of the operations that has been of concern to the gynecologic surgeon contemplating performance of a vaginal hysterectomy. A review of the literature, however, reveals that a reasonably large number of these patients have successfully undergone vaginal hysterectomy without untoward morbidity. This literature groups a variety of uterine suspension types together. Ventral fixation of the uterus to the anterior abdominal wall has been the occasional source of failure to complete a hysterectomy vaginally. Although in more recent years it would be uncommon to see a patient who has had this operation, it is sometimes recognized by applying traction to the cervix and noting dimpling of the anterior abdominal wall. The uterus has been noted by some authors to become tubular and attenuated, reaching from the abdominal wall to a prolapsed state low in the vagina. Some of these uteri have been removed transvaginally by applying traction to the point of fixation on a lax anterior abdominal wall and pulling it into the operative field. In a few patients the operation was accomplished mainly transvaginally but required a small abdominal incision to release the uterine fundus.

Cesarean Section

The patient who has undergone one and especially several cesarean sections is of concern to the gynecologic surgeon contemplating a vaginal hysterectomy. Several of the studies on previous pelvic surgery and vaginal hysterectomy contain small numbers of such patients. In the study by Coulam and Pratt,[2] 56 of the patients had undergone previous cesarean section. The chief concern in these patients centers on the difficulty of gaining entry into the scarred anterior cul-de-sac and the potential for bladder injury. Coulam and Pratt noted marked scarring from the previous cesarean section in some cases, but they successfully completed the vaginal hysterectomy in each case without incurring an injury. In two other studies, a combined total of 13 patients had undergone vaginal hysterectomy without incident after multiple prior cesarean sections.

Bladder injury is reported occasionally in these patients. To a variable degree the bladder becomes scarred to the cervix and lower uterine fundus. A greater amount of sharp dissection is therefore generally required to mobilize the bladder and gain entry into the anterior cul-de-sac. A number of methods have been recommended to facilitate this entry.

Continuous traction on the cervix and, at 45 degrees to this point, on the vaginal mucosa of the bladder flap facilitates sharp dissection. A cautious but firm pushing technique with the closed blunt tip of heavy Mayo scissors usually enables the surgeon to find the correct path of dissection (see Fig. 2-4). In the presence of dense fibrosis careful scissor dissection is required (Fig. 8-1). Frequent palpation under the bladder flap for the Foley balloon and inspection for a bluish tint of the tissues may also be helpful.

Filling or placing a probe in the bladder may be useful. Placing a finger or bent uterine sound around the uterine fundus from the posterior cul-de-sac (which can generally only be done with descensus and a normal size uterus) may guide the surgeon along the correct path of dissection (Figs. 8-2, 8-3, 8-4). Sharp dissection is carried underneath the finger or the tip of the sound until the tip can be seen through the tissue folds and the cul-de-sac entered.

Nichols and Randall[3] recommended that 30 ml of diluted indigo carmine, methylene blue, or sterile evaporated milk be instilled into the bladder preoperatively and be left in place during vaginal hyster-

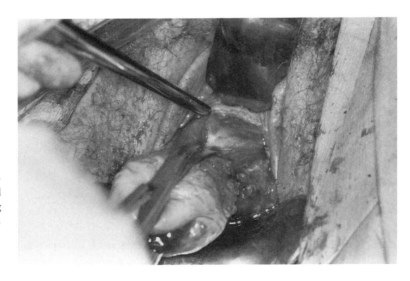

Figure 8-1. Sharp scissor dissection of a densely adherent bladder off the cervix and lower uterus. Note the strong outward and dorsal retraction of the cervix and exposure, and the countertraction with Deaver and smooth forceps.

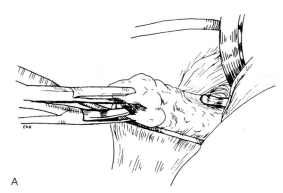

A

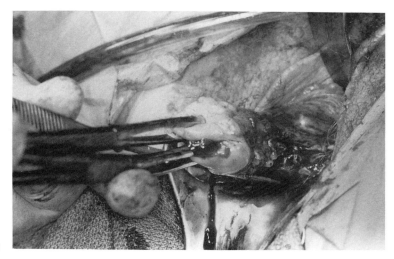

Figure 8-2. (A–C) A bent uterine sound has been placed through the posterior cul-de-sac and around the top of the broad ligament, with the tip pushing into the anterior cul-de-sac. With careful sharp dissection *underneath* the sound tip, a clear path can be found under the bladder into the anterior cul-de-sac.

B

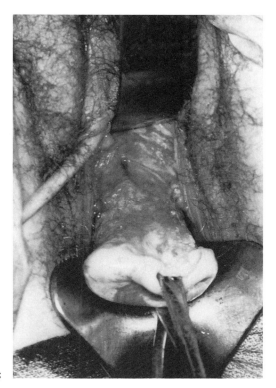

C

Figure 8-3. Tip of the sound is protruding through the safely made anterior culdotomy.

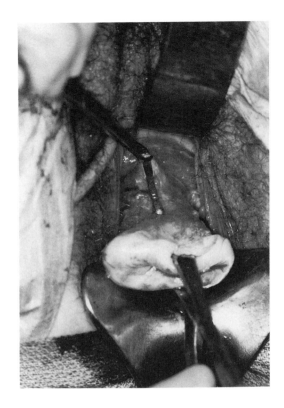

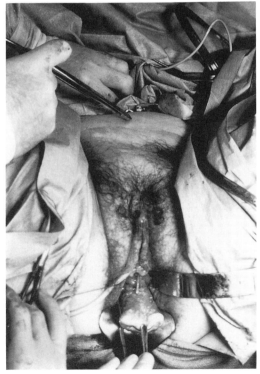

Figure 8-4. Uterine sound technique being utilized in an obese patient who had undergone three prior cesarean sections. The forceps handle points to the abdominal scar. Despite having had no prior vaginal births, there was considerable uterine descensus. A small struggle vaginally to avoid laparotomy may be of considerable benefit to such a patient. In fact, sometimes abdominal hysterectomy is considerably more of a struggle.

ectomy. With dilute methylene blue the operator should be able to visualize a bluish color through the tissue before an injury has occurred if dissecting close to the bladder and should immediately note it when a cystotomy is made.

Of considerable relevance is the opinion of several of the above investigators that dissection of the bladder from the cervix and uterus and avoidance of injury in such patients is not any easier from the abdominal approach.

Myomectomy

Some of the reports contain a few patients who had previously undergone myomectomy with no unusual difficulties noted with vaginal hysterectomy. Depending on the location of the myoma, the surgeon might expect a few adhesions of the omentum or intestine or perhaps some scarring of the anterior or posterior cul-de-sac.

Cul-de-sac Obliteration

An operation that would likely cause some difficulty when gaining entry into the posterior cul-de-sac would be a Moschowitz or Halban type obliteration of the posterior cul-de-sac. The difficulty would be encountered in this area after such procedures regardless of the route of hysterectomy. When operating transvaginally, great caution is warranted in the approach to the posterior cul-de-sac.

Surgical Considerations

As with other potentially difficult types of vaginal hysterectomy, the final decision as to the route of the hysterectomy is best made during the examination under anesthesia. It is especially important that the uterus is freely mobile. As an initial diagnostic step, a posterior culdotomy can be performed that allows the surgeon to better assess the anatomic alterations that may have occurred as a result of the previous surgery. With the posterior culdotomy, release of the lower ligaments may allow the surgeon greater access to make this assessment. As discussed above, in certain patients it is important to approach entry into the peritoneal cavity carefully. Careful examination under anesthesia may give the surgeon some idea as to the condition of the posterior cul-de-sac. In such patients the posterior cervical vaginal mucosa is incised, and the soft tissue including the peritoneum is mobilized off the back of the uterus. It may be helpful during this operation to proceed with ligation of the lower ligaments, as it would allow the surgeon access higher on the back of the uterus. Incising the vaginal mucosa in the midline and mobilizing the vaginal flaps laterally may also facilitate exposure and orient the surgeon as to the location of the rectum.

Through the posterior culdotomy the surgeon assesses the presence and nature of uterine adhesions, which are generally from the omentum, adnexa, sigmoid colon or epiploica, small intestine, or anterior abdominal wall. Extensive bowel adhesions with only limited involvement of the uterus is often better handled transvaginally. The transvaginal approach to such adhesions provides good exposure and avoids the extensive manipulation and dissection of the bowel that might well be necessary when operating transabdominally. The condition of the anterior cul-de-sac should also be assessed with the index finger if possible. Adhesions that are on the back of the uterus in clear view may be lysed at this time. The surgeon need be concerned only with adhesions that will interfere with safe ligation of the pedicles and removal of the uterus. Adhesions must be taken down only as they are encountered during progression of the hysterectomy to ensure maximum exposure.

Once the surgeon has assessed the situation through the posterior culdotomy and has determined that it is reasonable to proceed with the vaginal approach, entry should be gained into the anterior cul-de-sac. If the surgeon is concerned about the condition of the posterior cul-de-sac or was unsuccessful in gaining entry posteriorly, anterior culdotomy may be undertaken at an early stage. As discussed, in certain patients dissection of the bladder off the cervix and lower uterus and entry into the anterior cul-de-sac may be difficult. Often in such patients, however, the anterior cul-de-sac is entered without difficulty. If difficulty is encountered owing to obliteration of the surgical plane and scarring, sharp dissection is used with the aid of the previously described techniques.

Once entry is gained into the anterior and posterior cul-de-sacs and the uterine artery pedicles are ligated, adhesiolysis is facilitated. There is now access to the adhesions from both cul-de-sacs, and the uterus should be mobile, allowing the fundus to be pulled to or through either cul-de-sac, thereby giving excellent additional exposure to the adhesions. The uterus may also be morcellated if necessary at this point. Morcellation of the uterus sometimes facilitates exposure to adhesions. The hysterectomy is then completed, and the adnexae are assessed for possible removal.

Certain types of previous surgery and scarring may make transvaginal adnexectomy more difficult. On the other hand, a previously known disease process that has affected the adnexa, as discussed in Chapter 3, may make adnexectomy more important. However, when choosing to operate transvaginally, the surgeon should be primarily concerned with removing the uterus. Exposure to the adnexa is less adequate and difficult transvaginal removal of adnexa, as when extensively involved with a benign disease process or postsurgical distortion, is generally not necessary.

References

1. Campbell ZB. A report on 2,798 vaginal hysterectomies. Am J Obstet Gynecol 52:598–613, 1946
2. Coulam CB, Pratt JH. Vaginal hysterectomy: is previous pelvic operation a contraindication? Am J Obstet Gynecol 116:252–260, 1973
3. Nichols DH, Randall CL. Vaginal surgery (3rd ed). Maryland. Williams & Wilkins, Baltimore, 1989, p 186

Suggested Reading

Banks AL, Rutherford RN. Vaginal hysterectomy; individual variations in technic and end-results. West J Surg 63:23–30, 1955

Benson RC. Surgical complications of vaginal hysterectomy. Surg Gynecol Obstet 106:527–535, 1958

Bradford WZ, Bradford WB, Woltz JHE, Brown CW. Experiences with vaginal hysterectomy. Am J Obstet Gynecol 68:640–548, 1954

Brill HM, Golden M. Hysterectomy, the treatment of choice for benign enlargement of the uterus. Am J Obstet Gynecol 62:528–538, 1951

Carpenter RJ, Silva P. Vaginal hysterectomy following pelvic operation. Obstet Gynecol 30:394–398, 1967

Copenhaver EH. Vaginal hysterectomy: an analysis of indication and complications among 1,000 operations. Am J Obstet Gynecol 84:123–128, 1962

Counseller VS. Vaginal hysterectomy: indications, advantages, and surgical technic. Obstet Gynecol 1:84–93, 1953

Duckett HC, Williams JB Jr. Vaginal hysterectomy after previous surgery. J Fla Med Assoc 50:282–283, 1963

Falk HC, Bunkin IA. A study of 500 vaginal hysterectomies. Am J Obstet Gynecol 52:623–630, 1946

Gray LA. Vaginal Hysterectomy, Charles C Thomas, Springfield, IL, 1955, pp 47–48

Heaney NS. Vaginal hysterectomy—its indications and technique. Am J Surg 48:284–288, 1940

Hoffman MS, Jeager M. A new method for gaining entry into the scarred anterior cul-de-sac during transvaginal hysterectomy. Am J Obstet Gynecol 162:1269–1270, 1990

Ingram JM, Withers RW, Wright HL. Vaginal hysterectomy after previous pelvic surgery. Am J Obstet Gynecol 74:1181–1186, 1957

Isaacs JH. Vaginal hysterectomy. In Sciarra JJ, Droegemueller W (eds). Gynecology and Obstetrics (vol 1). Lippincott, Philadelphia, 1990, p 1

Israel SL. Vaginal sequelae of vaginal hysterectomy. Am J Obstet Gynecol 69:87–93, 1955

Jacobs WM, Rogers SF, Scheihing WC, Adels MJ. Advisability of vaginal hysterectomy after previous pelvic operations. J Int Coll Surg 34:196–199, 1960

Kaser O, Iklé FA, Hirsch HA. In Friedman EA (ed). Vaginal hysterectomy and vaginal procedures for uterine descensus. Atlas of Gynecologic Surgery (2nd ed). Thieme-Stratton, New York, 1985

Leventhal ML, Lazarus ML. Total abdominal and vaginal hysterectomy, a comparison. Am J Obstet Gynecol 61:289–299, 1951

Porges RF. Changing indications for vaginal hysterectomy. Am J Obstet Gynecol 136:153–158, 1980

Porges RF. Vaginal hysterectomy at Bellevue Hospital: an experience in teaching residents, 1963–1967. Obstet Gynecol 35:300–313, 1970

Rosenzweig BA, Seifer DB, Grant WD, et al. Urologic injury during vaginal hysterectomy: a case-central study. J Gynecol Surg 6:27–32, 1990

Wheelock JB, Krebs HB, Hurt WG. Sparing and repairing the bladder during gynecologic surgery. Contemp Obstet Gynecol 28:163–171, 1984

9

Miscellaneous Conditions

There are no doubt circumstances complicating vaginal hysterectomy that have not been covered in this book. Some miscellaneous conditions are included in this chapter for the sake of completeness. For purposes of a future edition, suggestions for additional coverage would be most appreciated.

Intraepithelial neoplasia of the cervix occasionally extends onto the vaginal fornix. Recognition of this condition and technical aspects of treatment with hysterectomy are reviewed.

Treatment of a prolapsed uterine leiomyoma may include myomectomy or hysterectomy. Timing and technical aspects of hysterectomy are discussed.

The standard (conventional) treatment for early endometrial cancer is abdominal hysterectomy with bilateral salpingo-oophorectomy. In highly individualized cases, however, vaginal hysterectomy is appropriate treatment. The literature and circumstances concerning vaginal hysterectomy for endometrial cancer are reviewed. The role of laparoscopy is also discussed.

Carcinoma In Situ of the Cervix and Vaginal Fornix

Carcinoma in situ of the cervix is an accepted indication for vaginal hysterectomy in the patient who has completed childbearing. The hysterectomy is performed in a straightforward manner with careful attention to the technique of vaginal cuff closure. Carcinoma in situ of the cervix is common, with approximately 50,000 new cases diagnosed each year. Carcinoma in situ of the vagina, on the other hand, is uncommon, accounting for approximately 0.4% of lower genital tract intraepithelial neoplasia. This disease most commonly is multifocal and involves the upper vagina. Many patients have already undergone a prior hysterectomy, most commonly for carcinoma in situ of the cervix. The lesions are usually detected during investigation of an abnormal Papanicolaou smear. The frequency of carcinoma in situ of the cervix coexisting with carcinoma in situ of the vagina is not known, but it appears from most reports to be uncommon. The above factors suggest that at least some of these vaginal lesions were missed at the time of prior evaluation and hysterectomy.

Careful colposcopic assessment of the vagina, especially the fornices, is warranted in patients undergoing evaluation for cervical carcinoma in situ. When carcinoma in situ also involves the fornix, it is reasonable to incorporate excision of this area into the vaginal hysterectomy. The vaginal area to be excised should be carefully demarcated, preferably colposcopically, with a planned 1 cm margin. The planned vaginal margin is incised and the involved vaginal mucosa undermined and mobilized to the cervix (Fig. 9-1). Submucosal infiltration with a vasoconstrictor facilitates this maneuver. The hysterectomy then proceeds in a standard fashion.

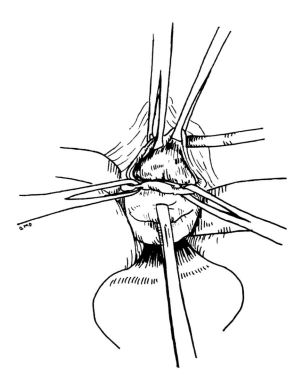

Figure 9-1. Portion of the anterior vaginal fornix involved with carcinoma in situ has been circumscribed and dissected off the bladder toward the cervix. Vaginal hysterectomy may now proceed in a routine manner, which will include removal of this portion of involved vaginal mucosa.

Vaginal shortening may be noted initially after any hysterectomy. With intercourse the vagina generally stretches back to a normal length within a few weeks. If it appears that the amount of vagina excised may result in significant shortening, the cuff should be left open and the cut edge sutured with interrupted or figure-of-eight stitches. A dilator is then placed, which requires intermittent use for some time. A short course of vaginal estrogen may aid in reepithelialization.

As with a hysterectomy for cervical carcinoma in situ, when the vaginal cuff is to be closed there must be careful attention to the technique. If possible, the mucosal edges should be inverted into the vagina. Areas of buried vaginal cuff mucosa may later develop into neoplastic vaginal cuff inclusion cysts, which are often difficult to detect.

When there is vaginal carcinoma in situ beyond the fornices, excision may leave a vagina of inadequate length for intercourse. Multiple colposcopically directed biopsies followed by laser vaporization of the vaginal disease provides a better functional result in such patients. Hysterectomy may be performed at that time or, preferably, after the vagina has healed.

Prolapsed Myoma

Occasionally a patient presents with cramping, a discharge, or irregular bleeding; and at pelvic examination a myoma is found prolapsed through the cervical os. Such myomas have usually lost much of their blood supply and are somewhat necrotic, ulcerated, and infected (Fig. 9-2). They can generally be excised transvaginally with little difficulty. With antibiotic coverage and anesthesia the dilated and effaced cervix is retracted laterally and upward, exposing the stalk of the myoma, which is then ligated (Fig. 9-3). If the myoma originates in the fundus, a tonsil snare can be used to cut the stalk near its base.

When it is the gynecologic surgeon's judgment that the patient would be best treated by hysterectomy, this operation may be performed at the same time or at a later date. Some reports have suggested that a two-stage approach to myomectomy and hysterectomy decreases infectious morbidity. With modern antibiotic usage a single-stage procedure usually works well. Treatment with a broad-spectrum antibiotic both before and after the operation is indicated in either case.

Once the myoma is removed, the previously expanded cervix returns to its normal size, safely distancing it from the ureters and giving the surgeon room to operate. The hysterectomy then proceeds in a standard fashion.

Figure 9-2. Large prolapsed myoma. Note the
resultant markedly increased
cervical diameter.

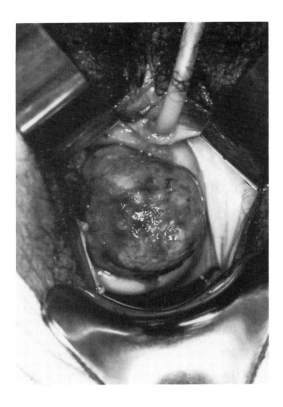

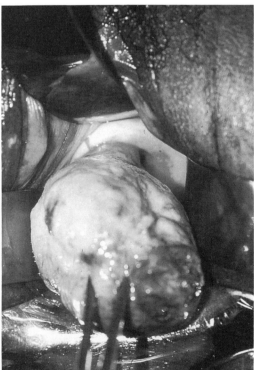

Figure 9-3. Traction on a
prolapsed submucous
myoma, exposing the stalk.

Stage I Endometrial Cancer

The standard treatment for early stage endometrial carcinoma is total abdominal hysterectomy with bilateral salpingo-oophorectomy. Unlike cancer of the cervix, the cure rate for endometrial carcinoma with radiotherapy alone is inferior to that of hysterectomy. Lymph node sampling is appropriate in selected patients, such as those with less well differentiated tumors, deep myometrial invasion, or lower uterine segment involvement identified on frozen section. Patients with positive lymph nodes or other high risk factors may benefit from postoperative adjuvant pelvic radiotherapy. Other types of adjuvant therapy may be offered in the event of carcinomatosis or positive peritoneal washings. Patients who would not tolerate surgery or who have locally advanced cancer are treated with radiotherapy.

A large proportion of patients with endometrial carcinoma are markedly obese, are in an older age group, and have many medical problems. Abdominal surgery in some of these patients has the potential for creating morbidity. Particularly in these patients, vaginal hysterectomy has been shown to produce less morbidity. For the medically compromised patient, the surgeon must judge the benefit of assessing the remainder of the abdominal cavity and retroperitoneal lymph nodes, as well as reliable removal of the adnexae, against the greater risk of abdominal surgery.

Certain factors can be used to select the patient who may be better served by a vaginal hysterectomy. Conditions such as morbid obesity and severe chronic obstructive pulmonary disease make the vaginal approach clearly more desirable than abdominal surgery, providing of course that the patient is otherwise a good candidate for a vaginal hysterectomy. Certain tumor factors can be identified preoperatively that make spread of the cancer outside the uterus much less likely. Such factors include well differentiated cancer, especially when it is found only focally on the curettage specimen, and a uterine fundus that is not obviously expanded. Transvaginal ultrasonography or perhaps magnetic resonance imaging to assess the depth of myometrial invasion and the adnexal pathology, hysteroscopic assessment of tumor size and location, and a serum CA-125 level are investigational methods that may also be useful in the future for helping to make this decision.

As with some of the other situations discussed in this book, the final decision as to the approach of the hysterectomy may be best made after the examination under anesthesia. The surgeon as usual assesses whether the anatomy lends itself well to a vaginal hysterectomy. It should be reasonably clear that morcellation will not be required. With experience the gynecologic surgeon can note some findings on examination that suggest the possibility of more significant disease. A cervix that is expanded or contains a gross lesion, the presence of parametrial shortening or nodularity, cul-de-sac nodularity, adnexal enlargement, marked uterine enlargement, or a separate pelvic side wall mass are highly significant findings that strongly suggest the possibility of a more advanced cancer. Vaginal hysterectomy is inappropriate for such patients. More subtle findings, such as a slightly enlarged, nodular, or unusually softened uterine fundus or an expanded lower uterine segment may also indicate the presence of high risk features such as deep myometrial invasion, a large tumor volume, or lower uterine segment involvement.

Each case must be individualized as to what treatment approach is in the patient's best interest. Considering the complexities involved in the infrequent selection of vaginal hysterectomy for the treatment of endometrial carcinoma, it is wise to make this decision in consultation with a gynecologic oncologist.

Many of the reports in the literature on vaginal hysterectomy include a small number of patients with a diagnosis of endometrial carcinoma. The opinion of these authors as well as other leading gynecologic surgeons is that vaginal hysterectomy is appropriate for endometrial carcinoma in highly selected cases. A review of the studies containing large numbers of patients who underwent vaginal hysterectomy for endometrial carcinoma, which includes a combined total of 960 patients, reveals that survival is comparable to other forms of treatment for stage I disease. Some of the patients in these series also received radiotherapy.

Several small studies have been published reporting on laparoscopy-assisted vaginal hysterectomy with laparoscopic lymphadenectomy for patients with early endometrial cancer. The advantages of the approach in certain operators' hands have been discussed in Chapter 3. Compared with the adbominal approach, the advantages of the laparoscopy-assisted vaginal hysterectomy include reduced morbidity and recovery time, the ability to assess the peritoneal cavity and lymph nodes, and greater ability to remove the adnexae. In endometrial cancer patients, however, the approach is limited by the frequently associated obesity or cardiopulmonary disease. Certain patients with early endometrial cancer and other medical problems may benefit from the laparoscopic approach. Currently the laparoscopic technique for the treatment of endometrial cancer is considered investigational.

Vaginal hysterectomy for carcinoma of the endometrium is performed in a straightforward manner. It is not necessary to purposefully include removal of a vaginal cuff with the cervix. Upon entering the posterior cul-de-sac, pelvic washings may be obtained. The surgeon should attempt to place the clamps along the sides of the cervix and uterine fundus so as to perform an extrafascial hysterectomy. The adnexae should also be removed if possible. The surgeon can consider the option of sending the uterus for frozen section after removal to detect the potential presence of high risk factors such as deep myometrial invasion, lower uterine segment involvement, or a poorly differentiated tumor. This information is useful only if the surgeon is planning to perform a laparotomy in the event of such findings. More commonly, when such high risk factors are found in the uterus after vaginal hysterectomy, consideration is given to postoperative adjuvant radiotherapy.

Suggested Reading

Carcinoma In Situ of the Cervix and Vaginal Fornix

Audet-Lapointe P, Body G, Vauclair R, Drovin P, Ayoub J. Vaginal intraepithelial neoplasia. Gynecol Oncol 36:232–239, 1990

Benedet JL, Sanders BH. Carcinoma in situ of the vagina. Am J Obstet Gynecol 148:695–700, 1984

Cancer Facts and Figures—1989. American Cancer Society, Atlanta, 1989

Capen CV, Masterson BJ, Magrina JF, Calkins JW. Laser therapy of vaginal intraepithelial neoplasia. Am J Obstet Gynecol 142:973–976, 1982

Copenhaver EH. Vaginal hysterectomy: an analysis of indication and complications among 1,000 operations. Am J Obstet Gynecol 84:123–128, 1962

Cramer D, Cutler S. Incidence and histopathology of malignancies of the female genital organs in the United States. Am J Obstet Gynecol 118:443–460, 1974

Curtin JP, Twiggs LB, Julian TM. Treatment of vaginal intraepithelial neoplasia with the CO_2 laser. J Reprod Med 30:942–944, 1985

Gallup DG, Morley G. Carcinoma in situ of the vagina. Obstet Gynecol 46:334–340, 1975

Geelhoed GW, Henson DE, Taylor PT, Ketcham AS. Carcinoma in situ of the vagina following treatment for carcinoma of the cervix: a distinctive clinical entity. Am J Obstet Gynecol 124:510–516, 1976

Hoffman MS, DeCesare SL, Roberts WS, et al. Upper vaginectomy for in-situ and occult superficially invasive carcinoma of the vagina. Am J Obstet Gynecol 166:30–33, 1992

Hoffman MS, Roberts WS, LaPolla JP, Fiorica FV, Cavanagh D. Laser vaporization of vaginal intraepithelial neoplasia III. Am J Obstet Gynecol

Hoffman MS, Roberts WS, LaPolla JP, Sterghos S Jr, Cavanagh D. Neoplasia in vaginal cuff inclusion cysts after hysterectomy. J Reprod Med 34:412–414, 1989

Isaacs JH. Vaginal hysterectomy. In Sciarra JJ, Droegemueller W (eds). Gynecology and Obstetrics (Vol 1). Lippincott, Philadelphia, 1990, p 2

Jimerson GK, Merrill JA. Cancer and dysplasia of the post-hysterectomy vaginal cuff. Gynecol Oncol 4:328–334, 1976

Jobson VW, Homesley HD. Treatment of vaginal intraepithelial neoplasia with the carbon dioxide laser. Obstet Gynecol 62:90–93, 1983

Krebs HB. Treatment of vaginal intraepithelial neoplasia with laser and topical 5-fluorouracil. Obstet Gynecol 73:657–660, 1989

Lenehan PM, Meffe F, Lickrish GM. Vaginal intraepithelial neoplasia: biologic aspects and management. Obstet Gynecol 68:333–337, 1986

Masterson BJ. Manual of Gynecologic Surgery. (2nd ed). Springer, New York, 1986, p 109

Petrilli ES, Townsend DE, Morrow CP, Nakao C. Vaginal intraepithelial neoplasia: biologic aspects and treatment with topical 5-fluorouracil and the carbon dioxide laser. Am J Obstet Gynecol 138:321–328, 1980

Stafl A, Wildinson EJ, Mattingly RF. Laser treatment of cervical and vaginal neoplasia. Am J Obstet Gynecol 128:136, 1977

Stuart GCE, Flagler EA, Nation JG, Dugan M, Robertson DI. Laser vaporization of vaginal intraepithelial neoplasia. Am J Obstet Gynecol 158:240–243, 1988

Townsend DE, Levine RV, Crum CP, Richard RM. Treatment of vaginal carcinoma in situ with the carbon dioxide laser. Am J Obstet Gynecol 143:565–568, 1982

Woodman CBJ, Jordan JA, Wade-Evans T. The management of vaginal intraepithelial neoplasia after hysterectomy. Br J Obstet Gynaecol 91:707–711, 1984

Prolapsed Myoma

Ben-Baruch G, Schiff E, Menashe Y, Menczer J. Immediate and late outcome of vaginal myomectomy for prolapsed pedunculated submucous myoma. Obstet Gynecol 72:858–861, 1988

Brooks GG, Stage AH. The surgical management of prolapsed pedunculated submucous leiomyomas. Surg Gynecol Obstet 141:397–398, 1975

Dicker D, Feldberg D, Dekel A, et al. The management of prolapsed submucous fibroids. Aust NZ J Obstet Gynaecol 26:308–311, 1986

Goldrath MH. Vaginal removal of the pedunculated submucous myoma: historical observations and development of a new procedure. J Reprod Med 35:921–924, 1990

Goldrath MH. Vaginal removal of the pedunculated submucous myoma: the use of Laminaria. Obstet Gynecol 70:670–672, 1987

Mattingly RF, Thompson JD. TeLinde's Operative Gynecology (6th ed). Lippincott, Philadelphia, 1985, p 219

Riley P. Treatment of prolapsed submucous fibroids. S Afr Med J 62:22–24, 1982

Sheth SS, Shinde L. Vaginal hysterectomy for myomatous polyp. J Gynecol Surg 9:101–103, 1993

Stage I Endometrial Cancer

Bloss JD, Berman ML, Bloss LP, Buller RE. Use of vaginal hysterectomy for the management of stage I endometrial cancer in the medically compromised patient. Gynecol Oncol 40:74–77, 1991

Cacciatore B, Lehtovirta P, Wahlström T, Ylöstalo P. Preoperative sonographic evaluation of endometrial cancer. Am J Obstet Gynecol 160:133–137, 1989

Candiani GB, Belloni C, Maggi R, et al. Evaluation of different surgical approaches in the treatment of endometrial cancer at FIGO stage I. Gynecol Oncol 37:6–8, 1990

Candiani GB, Mangioni C, Marzi MM. Surgery in endometrial cancer: age, route, and operability rate in 854 stage I and II fresh consecutive cases: 1955–76. Gynecol Oncol 6:363–372, 1978

Cassia LJS, Weppelmann B, Shingleton H, et al. Management of early endometrial carcinoma. Gynecol Oncol 35:362–366, 1989

Chen SS, Rumancik WM, Spiegel G. Magnetic resonance imaging in stage I endometrial carcinoma. Obstet Gynecol 75:274–277, 1990

Childers J, Surwit E, Hatch K. Laparoscopically assisted staging surgery (LASS) and vaginal hysterectomy (LAVH) for endometrial cancer [abstract]. Gynecol Oncol 49:110–111, 1993

Childers JM, Surwit EA. Combined laparoscopic and vaginal surgery for the management of two cases of stage 1 endometrial cancer. Gynecol Oncol 45:46–51, 1992

Conte M, Guariglia L, Benedetti-Panici P, et al. Transvaginal ultrasound evaluation of myometrial invasion in endometrial carcinoma. Gynecol Obstet Invest 29:224–226, 1990

DiSaia PJ, Creasman WT, Baronow RC, Blessing JA. Risk factors and recurrent patterns in stage I endometrial cancer. Am J Obstet Gynecol 151:1009–1015, 1985

Donato DM. Advanced laparoscopic techniques in gynecologic oncology. Contemp Obstet Gynecol September:102–118, 1992

Falk HC, Bunkin IA. A study of 500 vaginal hysterectomies. Am J Obstet Gynecol 52:623–630, 1946

Foley K, Lee RB. Surgical complications of obese patients with endometrial carcinoma. Gynecol Oncol 39:1711–1174, 1990

Gordon AN, Fleischer AC, Reed GW. Depth of myometrial invasion in endometrial cancer: preoperative assessment by transvaginal ultrasonography. Gynecol Oncol 39:321–327, 1990

Hirai Y, Kaku S, Teshima H, et al. Use of angio computed tomography to evaluate extent of endometrial carcinoma. Gynecol Oncol 33:372–375, 1989

Ingiulla W, Cosmi EV. Vaginal hysterectomy for the treatment of cancer of the corpus uteri. Am J Obstet Gynecol 100:541–543, 1968

Ingram JM, Withers RW, Wright HL. The debated indications for vaginal hysterectomy. South Med J 51:869–872, 1958

Isaacs JH. Vaginal hysterectomy. In Sciarra JJ, Droegemueller W (eds). Gynecology and Obstetrics (Vol 1). Lippincott, Philadelphia, 1990, p 2

Käser O, Iklé FA, Hirsch HA. Friedman EA (eds). Atlas of Gynecologic Surgery (2nd ed). Thieme-Stratton, New York, 1985

Kucera H, Varra N, Weghaupt K. Benefit of external irradiation in pathologic stage I endometrial carcinoma: a prospective clinical trial of 605 patients who received postoperative vaginal irradiation and additional pelvic irradiation in the presence of unfavorable prognostic factors. Gynecol Oncol 38:99–104, 1990

Kudo R, Yamauchi O, Okazaki T, et al. Vaginal hysterectomy without ligation of the ligaments of the cervix uteri. Surg Gynecol Obstet 170:299–305, 1990

Lewandowski G, Torrisi J, Potkul RK, et al. Hysterectomy with extended surgical staging and radiotherapy versus hysterectomy alone and radiotherapy in stage I endometrial cancer: a comparison of complication rates. Gynecol Oncol 36:401–404, 1990

Lotocki RJ, Copeland LJ, DePetrillo AD, Muirhead W. Stage I endometrial carcinoma: treatment results in 835 patients. Am J Obstet Gynecol 146:141–144, 1983

Malviya VK, Deppe G, Malone JM Jr, Sundarseson AS, Lawrence WD. Reliability of frozen section examination in identifying poor prognostic indicators in stage I endometrial adenocarcinoma. Gynecol Oncol 34:299–304, 1989

Marchetti DL, Caglar H, Driscoll DL, Hreshchyshyn MM. Pelvic radiation in stage I endometrial adenocarcinoma with high-risk attributes. Gynecol Oncol 37:51–54, 1990

Marziale P, Atlante G, Pozzi M, Diatrallevi F, Iacovelli A. 426 Cases of stage I endometrial carcinoma: a clinicopathological analysis. Gynecol Oncol 32:278–281, 1989

Mencaglia L, Scarselli G, Tantini C. Hysteroscopic evaluation of endometrial cancer. J Reprod Med 29:701–704, 1984

Morrow CP, Bundy BN, Kurman RJ, et al. Relationship between surgical-pathological risk factors and outcome in clinical stage I and II carcinoma of the endometrium: a Gynecologic Oncology Group study. Gynecol Oncol 40:55–65, 1991

Peters WA, Andersen WA, Thornton N Jr, Morley GW. The selective use of vaginal hysterectomy in the management of adenocarcinoma of the endometrium. Am J Obstet Gynecol 146:285–291, 1983

Photopulos GT, Stovall TG, Summitt RL Jr. Laparoscopic-assisted vaginal hysterectomy, bilateral salpingo-oophorectomy and pelvic lymph node sampling for endometrial cancer. Gynecol Surg 8:91–94, 1992

Piver MS, Hempling RE. A prospective trial of postoperative vaginal radium/cesium for grade 1–2 less than 50% myometrial invasion in surgical stage I endometrial adenocarcinoma. Cancer 66:1133–1138, 1990

Piver MS, Yazigi R, Blumenson L, Tsukada Y. A prospective trial comparing hysterectomy plus vaginal radium, and uterine radium plus hysterectomy in stage I endometrial carcinoma. Obstet Gynecol 54:85–89, 1979

Porges RF. Changing indications for vaginal hysterectomy. Am J Obstet Gynecol 136:153–158, 1980

Pratt JH, Symmonds RE, Welch JS. Vaginal hysterectomy for carcinoma of the fundus. Am J Obstet Gynecol 88:1063–1071, 1964

Schink JC, Rademaker AW, Miller DS, Lurain JR. Tumor size in endometrial cancer. Cancer 67:2791–2794, 1991

Spirtos NM, Schlaerth JB, Spirtos TW, Kimball RE. Laparoscopic bilateral aortic and pelvic lymph node sampling: a new technique [abstract]. Gynecol Oncol 49:137–138, 1993

Sutton GP, Geisler HE, Stehman FB, et al. Features associated with survival and disease-free survival in early endometrial cancer. Am J Obstet Gynecol 160:1385–1393, 1989

Tasche LW. 1700 Vaginal hysterectomies in a general surgical practice. Minn Med 51:1705–1711, 1968

Torrisi JR, Barnes WA, Popescu G, et al. Postoperative adjuvant external-beam radiotherapy in surgical stage I endometrial carcinoma. Cancer 64:1414–1417, 1989

VanBoudwdijk Bastiaanse MA. Cancer of the body of the uterus. Br J Obstet Gynaecol 59:611–620, 1952

INDEX

A

Abdominal hysterectomy, 1–2
Adenomyosis, 57
Adhesions
    and descensus, 73–74
    uterine, evaluation of, 114
Adnexa
    management of, 23–34, 67
    prior surgery involving, and indication for
        vaginal hysterectomy, 109
Adnexectomy, 16, 24, 25–30
    transvaginal, 23
        effects of prior surgery, 114–15
    using an endoloop suture, 25
Antibiotics
    after rectal laceration repair, 45
    in uterine prolapse, with ulceration,
        83
Arteries
    iliac, ligation of anterior division, 51
    uterine, ligation of, 13, 17
Assistants
    qualifications of, 6

B

Bladder
    anterior fundus of, opening, 47
    injury to, after cesarean section, 109–10
    laceration of, complication, 40–44
    mobilizing off the cervix, 10–11, 33,
        85–88
    prolapsed, 83
    testing the integrity of, 40

C

Cancer
    endometrial, 121–23
    ovarian, oophorectomy for preventing,
        23–24
Carcinoma in situ, cervical, indication for
        vaginal hysterectomy, 117–19
Catheter
    Foley, 7, 103
        removal of, 104
        use after bladder repair, 44
        use after ureter repair, 47
    suprapubic, 47

Cervicectomy, 60
Cervix
    carcinoma in situ, 117–19
    hypertrophy of, 81
Cesarean section, 109–13
    and likelihood of bladder laceration, 40
Clamps
    Zeplin parametrium, 6–7, 74–75
Colpopexy, sacrospinous, 91–98, 99
Colporrhaphy, 20
    anterior, 91
        and ureteral injury, 46
        vaginal wall prolapse following,
            98–99
    posterior, 91
Colposuspension, 101, 103
Colpotomy, posterior incision, 57–58
    and lack of descensus, 74–75
Complications, intraoperative, 39–51
Cul-de-sac, 7–8
    anterior, 11–12, 75, 89
        assessment of, 114
        and bladder injury, 40
        scarring after cesarean section,
            109–10
    posterior, 44–45, 81, 88, 89
        examination under anesthesia, 113
        obliteration of, 89–90
        obliteration of, in prior surgery,
            113
        in uterine prolapse, 83
Culdoplasty
    McCall's stitch, 16, 19, 89–90, 99
    and ureteral injury, 46
Culdotomy
    anterior, 114
    posterior, diagnostic, 113
Cystectomy
    in hemorrhage, 49
    for an ovarian tumor, 33–34
Cystoscope, 103
Cystoscopy, 39
Cystotomy, 42, 113
Cysts
    functional, 33–34
    neoplastic, vaginal cuff inclusion, 119

D
Descensus, 54–55
    as a criterion for vaginal hysterectomy, 71
    lack of, 71–78
Dissection
    in four-corner needle suspension, 99–100
    and scarring from cesarean section, 110

E
Endoloop suture, 25–26, 31
Endometriosis
    and likelihood of bladder laceration, 40
    and likelihood of rectal laceration, 44
    possible prevention of, by oophorectomy,
        23–24
    surgery for, and vaginal hysterectomy,
        109
Enterocele, prevention of, 19, 89–90, 104
Epinephrine, to control bleeding, 7
Episiotomy, 73
Estrogen replacement therapy, preoperative,
    83
Examination
    under anesthesia, 6, 57, 73, 113
        evaluating endometrial cancer, 121–22

F
Fallopian tubes
    bleeding from, 48–49
    removal of, 24
Fibrosis, scissors dissection in the presence
    of, 110
Fornix, vaginal
    carcinoma in situ, 118–19
Four-corner needle suspension, 99–104

G
Genital tract defects, repair of, 81
Gonadotropin-releasing hormone agonist, for
    preoperative management of enlarged
    uteri, 67

H
Hemisection, uterine, 60, 63–65, 77–78
Hemorrhage, 48–51
    from fallopian tubes or ovary, 48–49

Hemostasis, 16
Historic background, 1–2
    removal of enlarged uteri, 53–54
Hydroureteronephrosis, with prolapsed
    uterus, 85

I

Incision
    Schuchardt, 73–74, 75–76
Incontinence, stress, 102–3
Indigo carmine
    for evaluating ureteral injury, 47, 103
    for identifying the bladder, 110, 113
Infundibulopelvic ligament
    hemorrhage in the area of, 48
    visualization of, 32
Instruments, 6–7, 24–25
    for management, in lack of descensus, 74–75
    for morcellation of the enlarged uterus, 56
    for sacrospinous colpopexy, 92
Intramyometrial coring, 60, 65–67

L

Laparoscopy, for assisting vaginal hyster-
    ectomy, 31–33, 73, 122
Laparotomy, 6, 48
    to manage repair of injuries during surgery,
    45, 47
Leiomyomas, and advisability of transvaginal
    hysterectomy, 55, 57
Levator plate, reinforcement of, 96
Ligaments
    broad, 13, 17, 24, 57, 63
        tear in, 48
    cardinal, 13, 74–75, 88
    infundibulopelvic, access to, 25, 30–31
    pubourethral, 100
    round, 24, 32–33
    uterosacral, 74–75
    vesicouterine, 13, 88–89
Lymphadenectomy, in endometrial cancer,
    122

M

Magnetic resonance imaging, for assessing
    endometrial cancer, 121

Malignancy, biopsy for, in uterine prolapse
    with ulceration, 83
Mesovarium, oophorectomy at the level of,
    25, 31
Methylene blue
    for detecting bladder injury, 40
    for identifying the bladder, 110, 113
Milk, for identifying the bladder, 110, 113
Miya hook, 92–94
Mobilization
    of the bladder, 10–11, 33, 85–88
Morbidity
    abdominal versus vaginal hysterectomy, 1
    laparotomy versus vaginal hysterectomy,
    53–54
    in surgery for prolapsed myoma, 119
Morcellation
    and adhesions, 114
    of enlarged uteri, 53
    during intramyometrial coring, 67
    ovarian, 34
    posterior fundal, 60–63
Multiparity, and uterine prolapse, 81, 83
Myomas
    prolapsed, 119–20
    and selection for transvaginal hysterectomy,
    55
    size reduction with gonadotropin-releasing
    hormone agonist, 67
Myomectomy, 59–60
    during posterior fundal morcellation, 63, 65
    prior, and vaginal hysterectomy, 113

N

Needle, Stamey, 101
Neoplasia, genital tract intraepithelial, 118. *See
    also* Cancer; Carcinoma
Neurosurgery headlight, 6–7

O

Obesity
    and endometrial cancer, 121
    and selection for transvaginal hysterectomy,
    55, 73, 121
Oophorectomy
    in hemorrhage, 49

Oophorectomy (*continued*)
mesovarium, 25, 31
prophylactic, 23–24, 25
to remove an ovarian tumor, 33–34
Ovarian cancer, oophorectomy for
preventing, 23–24
Ovarian tumors, unsuspected, 33–34
Ovary
bleeding from, 48
retained, syndrome, 24

P
Paravaginal defect, repair of, 98–99
Patients, selection of. *See* Selection, of patients
Pedicles
adnexal, ligation of, 66–67
cardinal ligament, 99, 100–101
infundibulopelvic ligament, 49
ligation of, with lack of descensus, 75–76
paracervical, 48
uterine-adnexal, 24
uterine artery, 54, 56–57, 77, 88, 114
utero-ovarian, 16–18
ligation of, 48–49
Pelvic inflammatory disease
and descensus, 73
and likelihood of bladder laceration, 40
and likelihood of rectal laceration, 44
surgery for, and vaginal hysterectomy,
109
Pelvic relaxation, as a criterion for vaginal
hysterectomy, 71
Perineorrhaphy, 91
Peritoneal defect, purse-string closure
of, 19
Peritoneal fold, anterior, 11–12
Plication
bladder neck, 102–3
cystocele, 102
urethrovesicle angle, 104
Polygalactic acid versus chromic, gut suture
material, 20
Position, dorsal lithotomy, for vaginal hysterectomy, 5–6
Prolapse
as a criterion for vaginal hysterectomy, 71

definitions of, 72
and ureteral injury, 46
uterine, as a criterion for vaginal hysterectomy, 81–105
Pseudoprolapse, 83

R
Reconstruction of support, prolapsed uterus,
84, 89–91
Recovery, time for, abdominal versus vaginal
hysterectomy, 2
Rectocele, repair of, 96, 104
Rectum
laceration of, 44–45
prolapsed, 83
Respiratory disease, chronic, and selection for
transvaginal hysterectomy, 55
Retained ovary syndrome, 24
Retractors
Breisky-Navratil, 92
Heaney, 6–7, 10–11

S
Sacrospinal ligament-coccygeus muscle
complex, 92
Salpingectomy, prophylactic, 24
Salpingo-oophorectomy
bilateral, 31–33
for endometrial carcinoma, 121–23
risks of, 24
selection of cases for, 48
Schuchardt incision, 73–74, 75–76
Scissors
Jorghenson, 6–7, 25
Mayo, 6–7, 74–75, 110
for intramyometrial coring, 67
Selection of patients, 54–56, 57
criteria for, 71–72
with prolapsed uterus, 85
Sigmoid colon, injury to, 45
Size
of the uterus, and choice of surgery, 54
Small bowel, laceration of, 45–46
Space of Retzius, 47, 99–100
Stitches
McCall's type culdoplasty, 16, 19, 89–90, 99

puborectalis plication, 96
"pulley", 96–97
transfixation type, 13
triple helical, 100
Support
    reconstruction of, in prolapsed uterus
        surgery, 84, 89–91
    urethral and rectal, 104
Supravaginal septum, 10
Surgery, prior, and indication for vaginal
        hysterectomy, 107–15
Suspension, uterine, and vaginal hyster-
        ectomy, 109
Suture
    absorbable, 13
      for vaginal closure, 103
    bladder neck, 100
    chromic, 43, 45
    polypropylene, 94, 96–97, 100
    purse-string
      of a peritoneal defect, 19
      for peritoneal defect closure, 89, 104–5
    for repairing a lacerated bladder, 42–43

T
Tumors
    ovarian, unsuspected, 33–34
    See also Cancer; Carcinoma; Malignancy

U
Ultrasonography
    for detecting ovarian tumors, 33–34

transvaginal, for assessing endometrial
    cancer, 121
Ureteroneocystostomy, to correct ureter
        injury, 47
Ureters
    injury to, 46–47
    prolapsed, 83
    visualization of, 32
Urethra, prolapsed, 83
Urinary tract, distortion of, with prolapsed
        uterus, 81
Urologic injuries, 39
Uteri
    enlarged, transvaginal removal of, 2,
      53–68
Uterosacral-cardinal ligament complex, 13–15
    and anatomic changes in the ureter, 46
    reattachment to the vaginal cuff, 81
    and support for the vaginal cuff, 89–90
    and uterine descensus, 74–75

V
Vagina
    anterior wall prolapse, 98–99
    effect of hysterectomy on, 119
Vaginal cuff
    closure of, 119
    reattachment of the uterosacral-cardinal
      ligament complex to, 81
Vaginectomy, 104–5
Vasopressin, to control back bleeding, 7
Vault, prevention of prolapse of, 89